THE

E   M   R

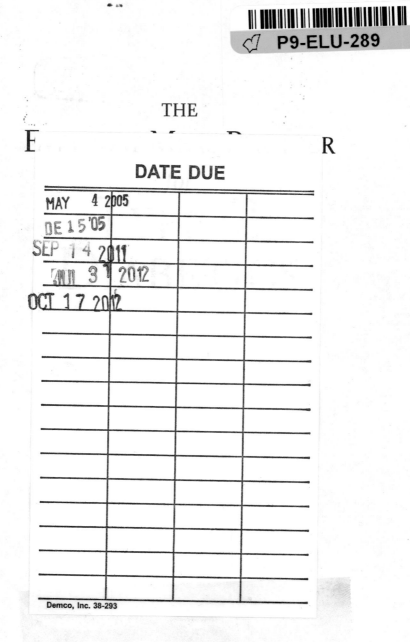

DATE DUE

MAY 4 2005		
DE 1 5 '05		
SEP 1 4 2011		
JAN 3 1 2012		
OCT 17 2012		

THE
EVERYDAY MEAL PLANNER
for
TYPE 2
DIABETICS

KRISTEN L. CARON, B.S., M.A., AND AARON HENRY

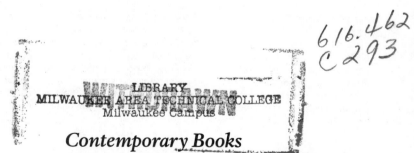

Contemporary Books

Chicago New York San Francisco Lisbon London Madrid Mexico City
Milan New Delhi San Juan Seoul Singapore Sydney Toronto

Library of Congress Cataloging-in-Publication Data

Caron, Kristen L.
    The everyday meal planner for type 2 diabetics : simple tips for healthy dining at home or on the town / by Kristen Caron and Aaron Henry.
       p.   cm.
    Includes bibliographical references and index.
    ISBN 0-7373-0554-1
     1. Non-insulin-dependent diabetes—Diet therapy.   2. Non-insulin-dependent diabetes—Diet therapy—Recipes.   I. Henry, Aaron.   II. Title.

RC662 .C36   2002
616.4′620654—dc21
                                                        2002019684

Contemporary Books

A Division of The McGraw·Hill Companies

2 3 4 5 6 7 8 9 0   DOC/DOC   1 0 9 8 7 6 5 4 3 2

ISBN 0-7373-0554-1

This book was set in Centaur by Lovedog Studio
Printed and bound by R. R. Donnelley—Crawfordsville

Cover design by Laurie Young
Cover photo: © FoodPix

McGraw-Hill books are available at special quantity discounts to use as premiums and sales promotions, or for use in corporate training programs. For more information, please write to the Director of Special Sales, Professional Publishing, McGraw-Hill, Two Penn Plaza, New York, NY 10121-2298. Or contact your local bookstore.

Important notice: The purpose of this book is to educate. It is sold with the understanding that the author and publisher shall have neither liability nor responsibility for any injury caused or alleged to be caused directly or indirectly by the information contained in this book. While every effort has been made to ensure its accuracy, the book's contents should not be construed as medical advice. Each person's health needs are unique. To obtain recommendations appropriate to your particular situation, please consult a qualified health care provider. Any herbal iinformation in this book is provided for education purposes only and is not meant to be used without consulting a qualified health practioner who is trained in herbal medicine.

This book is printed on acid-free paper.

Contents

Acknowledgments

We would like to give a special thank-you to our editor, L. Hudson Perigo. Her patience and guidance have proved invaluable time and time again. We would also like to thank the following persons for their contributions to the book: Rami Aizic, Mason Sommers, Dayla Frasier, and Carole Ghertner. To our friends and families, we thank you for lending your ears and offering wisdom and support. We appreciate you.

Introduction

The Everyday Meal Planner for Type 2 Diabetics is a comprehensive resource for individuals with Type 2 diabetes. While it is a book about functioning within your special dietary restrictions, it is not a *diet* book in that it provides no specific recommendations or formulas for weight loss. If you're seeking to lose weight, then the best use of this dining guide is in conjunction with a physician-guided weight loss program.

Losing weight in today's fast-paced, hectic world is not easy, especially when most of us are constantly on the go; we're surrounded by fast food eateries, and even the "diet" items in grocery stores can be labeled in ways that are misleading. The tools and information we provide can augment your weight loss program and help you achieve the goals you set for yourself.

We know how difficult it is for people with diabetes to meet their dietary needs, so we've created a book that does your meal planning for you—both in the home and away from home. This book provides tips for everything, from everyday meals, to dining in during the holidays, to dining out under special circumstances. We'll provide information on reading labels, grocery shopping, ordering from the menu at a variety of restaurants, and eating while traveling—whether you're on the road, in the air, or at sea. You'll be able to choose which method of controlling your diet works for you, using the information we provide.

Before we provide you with the tools to make your everyday dining experiences easier, let's take a look at the prevalence of diabetes. It is estimated that at least sixteen million people in the United States alone have diabetes. It is further estimated that half of all people with diabetes are *undiagnosed*. Of the diagnosed group, roughly 10 percent are those with Type 1 diabetes. Type 1 diabetes is defined as an absolute deficiency in insulin secretion. The onset of Type 1 diabetes is often at an early age, and may be the result of an autoimmune pathology, such as a virus. The remaining 90 percent of people with diabetes are classified as having Type 2 diabetes. Type 2 diabetes is caused by insulin resistance and/or inadequate insulin secretion. Of this group, the greater majority is clinically obese. Genetic predisposition also plays a strong role in the development of Type 2 diabetes.

The statistics become even more staggering when we look at the medical consequences of undiagnosed and/or untreated diabetes and untreated obesity. As we mentioned, there are an estimated sixteen million people with diabetes. Of this group, more than 80 percent are obese—possibly, even as high as 90 percent. Obesity is defined as being 20 percent over ideal body weight. Overweight adults (ages twenty to seventy-five) have a risk for developing diabetes that is 3 times greater than that of their ideal weight counterparts. Overweight adults have as high as a 2.1 times greater risk for having elevated cholesterol (this is estimated for those between the ages of twenty and forty-five). Even more astonishing, heart disease is 4 times more prevalent in the diabetic community.

If diabetes goes untreated, some very serious consequences can occur. Aside from the secondary medical conditions cited above, there are conditions that worsen with uncontrolled diabetes. There is damage to the eyes (retinopathy), the kidneys (nephropathy), the nerves (neuropathy), and the blood vessels. Elevated blood pressure, in addition to elevated triglycerides and cholesterol, is referred to as Syndrome X. This combination can be lethal for the heart. With this as a possible outcome, why should anyone choose to go untreated? You have the ability to get diagnosed, gather the information you need to maintain a lifestyle that addresses the special health needs of a person with diabetes, and make a change.

If you have picked up this book, you have, in all likelihood, already received a diagnosis of Type 2 diabetes. Perhaps you have worked with a dietitian or a diabetes educator. It is recommended that you continue to utilize these professionals for specific dietary recommendations. If you are uncertain as to whether or not you have diabetes, please seek out your physician for further diagnosis.

The first section of the book will provide different tools for selecting foods, including an explanation of the glycemic index, diabetes exchange lists, a full list of foods with respective carbohydrate counts, and a brief description of the American Diabetes Association (ADA) recommendations using the Food Guide Pyramid.

The tools we provide are designed to help you meet the health goals for people with diabetes as laid out by the ADA.

* Maintain as near-normal a blood glucose level as possible.
* Achieve optimal serum lipid levels (e.g., achieve normal levels of cholesterol and triglycerides).
* Achieve a healthy blood pressure level (e.g., lower than 140/80 mm/Hg).
* Maintain or attain a reasonable body weight.

Our aim is to simplify the dining experience for people with diabetes. With a few tools and food knowledge at your disposal, you should have no trouble coping with any dining situation that life throws your way, even when you're stressed or on the run. We encourage you to utilize all the information you'll find in this sourcebook to create the most beneficial and comfortable dining experience for you.

The food recommendations in this dining guide are based in part on the glycemic index, which we'll explain at length later. But for now, it's enough to know that the glycemic index is an index of values assigned to foods and indicates how much and how quickly these foods elevate your blood sugar levels. Generally, low glycemic foods are preferable to high glycemic foods, although we'll qualify this statement later with explanations of how fat plays a role in determining glycemic value, and why foods with a low glycemic value but high in fat should be avoided.

It is important to note early on that the research used to assign glycemic values to foods has shown that it is nearly impossible to predict, based on the carbohydrate content or other factors, whether certain foods will be high or low in glycemic value. Only rigorous testing determines the glycemic value; therefore, you should look at the glycemic chart for a particular food's glycemic value, instead of making assumptions on your own. Your expectations may be incorrect when you see how your favorite foods rank.

In addition to the glycemic index, we have incorporated the United States Department of Agriculture's Food Guide Pyramid—including modifications for the version revised for people with diabetes—and the American Diabetic Association's Exchange Lists into our dietary recommendations. The Food Guide Pyramid and Exchange Lists are helpful tools in maintaining a balanced diet.

The Food Guide Pyramid and the Exchange Lists are the commonly accepted standards for controlling dietary intake. The Food Guide Pyramid is not a diet; rather, it is a general guide to making sound dietary choices. There are modified pyramids designed to address specific needs. A Food Guide Pyramid for youth has been recently established.

The Exchange Lists are a tool used by individuals with diabetes to control the amount of carbohydrate consumed. Again, the list is not a diet in and of itself; it is a simple way to categorize foods in various groups by assigning an average carbohydrate content. This allows people with diabetes more control when choosing meals; with an understanding of carbohydrate content, individuals can effectively modify their intake.

Finally, we provide an extensive list derived from the USDA that lists foods and their nutrient content. Exchange lists give average numbers for carbohydrate content. The food list derived from USDA lists provides more specific numbers.

Although this may sound like a lot of information to sort through, we will make sense of it by providing specific dining guidelines that address all the important dietary considerations. The purpose of this book is to empower the reader in making dietary decisions. With the tools provided, you will have the ability to make educated choices.

Chapter One

Tools for Healthy Choices

. . . .

The Glycemic Index

The glycemic index is a list of foods ranked according to the rate at which they raise blood sugar levels. (See table I.I.) Thus, the index, which ranges from 0 to 100, can be a useful tool in selecting foods that are more likely to help you control your blood sugar. In practice, choosing foods from the lower end of the index will provide a more stable blood sugar. Conversely, foods at the high end create a rapid rise in blood sugar levels. Calvin Ezrin, M.D., a leading endocrinologist and co-author of *Your Fat Can Make You Thin*, provides the following explanation of the way in which glucagon and insulin are related to maintenance of blood sugar and weight.

Insulin and glucagon are the two major hormones made by the pancreas. They have opposite actions but normally act cooperatively to maintain a healthy balance of the major nutrients—protein, fat and carbohydrate. Insulin is the blood-sugar–lowering hormone, but other major actions are fat buildup and salt and water retention. Carbohydrate feeding stimulates the secretion of insulin and inhibits the release of glucagon. Low blood sugar increases glucagon output, which raises blood sugar rapidly to restore normal balance. (C. Ezrin and C. H. Best, "The Clinical and Metabolic Effects of Glucagon," *Canadian Medical Association Journal* 78, [1958]: 96–98.)

There are several factors that affect whether or not a food item creates a rapid, moderate, or low response in the rise of blood sugar. In this section, we'll discuss those factors. We'll also provide a brief list of foods with their glycemic index values. For a more extensive list of foods and a detailed explanation of the glycemic index, you can refer to *The Glucose Revolution: The Authoritative Guide to the Glycemic Index*, by Jennie Brand-Miller, Ph.D.; Thomas M. S. Wolever, M.D., Ph.D.; Stephen Colagiuri, M.D.; and Kaye Foster-Powell, M. Nutr. & Diet.

We should also note that the American Diabetes Association does not formally recognize the glycemic index as a dietary tool in the management of diabetes, because according to Brand-Miller et al., the ADA doesn't recognize the difference in blood sugar responses to different foods. They write, "An underlying assumption of the carbohydrate portions theory is the equivalent amounts of the carbohydrate, regardless of the type, cause an equal change in blood sugar level" (Brand-Miller et al., *The Glucose Revolution*, 105). This does not undermine the validity of the glycemic index. There are differing schools of thought on diabetic diets; however, the glycemic index utilizes what is arguably the most up-to-date and proven research.

In a study published in 1999, David S. Ludwig et al. demonstrated how the glycemic index has an effect on metabolism in obese persons. Subjects were fed meals that varied in overall glycemic values. Various outcomes were measured. Of those, for the purpose of this discussion, the outcome of increased calorie intake and elevated insulin levels is important.

It was found that subjects who consume meals with high glycemic index (G.I.) foods subsequently consume more calories after main meals. Hunger levels are perceptually higher after intake of high G.I. meals. The relationship, in simple terms, is that elevated insulin promotes glucose uptake in muscle and liver. This creates a drop in glucose levels, creating hunger to "restore" energy needs. Thus, higher G.I. diets exacerbate hunger while lower G.I. diets seem to keep hunger in check (David Ludwig, *Pediatrics* 103, no. 3 [March 1999]).

Some people with Type 2 diabetes produce an excess of insulin as a method of controlling blood sugar levels. If the body of a person with Type 2 diabetes does not properly utilize insulin, the resulting condition is known as hyperinsulinemia (elevated levels of insulin), which contributes to fat storage and increases the likelihood of obesity.

The glycemic index isn't a new craze; the index has been researched and tested for nearly thirty years. Gerald Reaven of Stanford Medical School is credited with early research on the glycemic index (*Science News*, 2000). More recently, researchers at Harvard Medical School have given attention to the index and its usefulness in the never-ending war against weight management. Researchers do generally agree that the index is straightforward for individuals without diabetes who make better use of the hormone insulin; however, this does not mitigate its usefulness for people with Type 2 diabetes.

Glycemic index use is simply another approach to dietary management, and most reputable approaches to dieting are in agreement that fat and carbohydrate intake must be controlled. We believe that the glycemic index is a useful tool, and should be considered in addition to other factors, such as carbohydrate amounts, when you're preparing meals. In this book, we've included both recommendations from the glycemic index and methods approved by the American Diabetes Association (that is, the Food Guide Pyramid and Exchange Lists) to give you comprehensive dietary guidelines.

Factors That Affect the Glycemic Value

Research suggests that the most important factor affecting glycemic value is the physical state of starch in foods. The less gelatinized (swollen) a starch is, the slower the rate of digestion. For example, the fibrous coat that surrounds beans and seeds creates a physical barrier that keeps the digestive enzymes from doing their job, thus slowing down the process of digestion. Consequently, many beans and seeds have a low glycemic value.

Cooking, the method of cooking, and combinations of food all impact the physical state of starch in the food. As your body's speed of digestion of the food is affected by its state, the glycemic values of the foods will change as well. For example, foods that have a certain glycemic value when boiled, such as potatoes, may suddenly acquire a high glycemic value after they're cooked and mashed. A food in its cooked state may be more quickly digested by your body, rapidly boosting your blood's sugar level. Consequently, the food may be given a higher glycemic value depending on its preparation.

How you combine foods when you consume them also affects the glycemic index. Numbers for glycemic values are determined by testing a specific sample weight of any given food. For example, a set amount of weight for white rice is tested to render a glycemic value, which is high. If white rice is consumed with a very low glycemic food, like lentils, the *total* glycemic value will be lower. The math gets tricky, but here's an illustration of how this might work in a meal.

Let's suppose you have a meal comprised of mashed potatoes, baked chicken, grilled vegetables, and salad. Let's further assume that you have equal amounts in carbohydrates of both vegetables (low glycemic index value) and mashed potatoes (high glycemic index value), e.g., 15 grams carbohydrate portions of each. You can then average the glycemic value of the foods to get a moderate glycemic value. (Remember: This assumes that you are consuming equal carbohydrate amounts of the foods.) The reality in most meal planning is that foods are eaten in combination. So while you might consume a food that has a high glycemic index number, the overall effect on blood sugar can be lowered if that food is consumed with a lower glycemic index food. For example, eating half a sandwich on one slice of white bread (high glycemic index value) can be counterbalanced with the turkey in your sandwich (low glycemic index value), as well as by also eating a dessert serving of cherries (low glycemic index value).

Fiber

Fiber is also a factor in determining glycemic value. It's believed that fibers decrease starch and enzyme interaction by increasing the viscosity of intestinal contents. The viscous state of the intestinal contents slows down the rate of digestion, so your blood sugar level is not elevated as dramatically or as quickly.

Fiber content can earn low glycemic values for foods that are "dessert" foods. For example, an oatmeal cookie, because of its fiber content, receives a lower glycemic value than a vanilla wafer that lacks fiber and is more rapidly digested by your system. Although both are cookies—and dessert foods—an oatmeal cookie is a better choice because its fiber content beneficially affects the way your body digests it.

As you look at our preplanned meals, and plan your own meals, try to introduce fiber into your diet. This can be done in a myriad of ways, such as eating a high-fiber cereal for breakfast, or using whole grain breads for your sandwiches.

The story of dietary fiber grows a little more complex. There are two different types of fiber, each of which functions in different ways to meet your dietary needs.

Insoluble fiber is fiber that does not break down into sugar in your body. Insoluble fibers eliminate toxins from your system and aid in digestion by assisting the passage of foods through the gut. Insoluble fibers are rich in cellulose, which regulates glucose and hemicellulose in the body. Lignin in insoluble fiber provides protection against colon cancer and gallstones. Lignin can absorb water. This type of fiber is helpful because it "swells," causing a feeling of fullness and making digestion easier by helping the intestine pass water. Insoluble fiber is found in a variety of foods such as fruits, vegetables, and wheat.

Soluble fiber aids in reducing blood cholesterol levels by "attaching" to by-products of cholesterol, such as bile acids, and helping to regulate the body's use of sugar. Pectin in soluble fiber lowers cholesterol. Sources of soluble fiber are dried beans and legumes, oat bran, and cornmeal.

Acid Content

The high acid content in foods like vinegar, sourdough bread, or lemon juice also slows down gastric emptying (the passage of food out of your stomach). By extension, this creates slower digestion of carbohydrates, resulting in lower elevation of your blood sugar levels. One way to introduce acid content into your foods is by using vinegars and acidic fruit juices, such as lemon juice, in cooking or in salads.

A simple salad dressing recipe that can boost the acid content in your diet is as follows: Add 2–3 tablespoons of vinegar (try white balsamic) to every 1 tablespoon of olive oil. Add a teaspoon of Dijon-type mustard and your favorite herbs; we suggest basil, tarragon, black pepper, and a touch of garlic.

Sugars

Contrary to what you might think, sucrose, or table sugar, doesn't create an instant rise in blood sugar. Sucrose is composed of one glucose molecule and one fructose molecule. Fructose is a low glycemic sugar; in other words, it slowly converts to glucose. The slow conversion to fructose means that your body digests sucrose more slowly, and your blood sugar level is not affected as rapidly as, for example, a serving of graham crackers or a slice of white bread.

This doesn't mean that we are suggesting you run out and grab loads of candy and cakes; only that products with sucrose are not strictly forbidden. It should be noted that there is no nutritional value in refined sugar. Eating sugar—in this case, sucrose—is fine as long as it is in small amounts and is *balanced* with other foods that provide adequate nutrients. We still recommend that sugar intake be reduced in the diabetic diet.

Many products contain the sugar maltose. The chemical structure of maltose is two glucose molecules. Avoid maltose, found in baked goods, ice cream, food supplements, and cereals, because it will rapidly raise your blood sugar levels.

Fruit sugar, or fructose, as mentioned above, has a lower glycemic value. Because of this, some fruits tend to be lower on the glycemic index. There is, however, a wide range of values. Some generalizations can be made. Orchard fruits, like apples, peaches, plums, cherries (think fruit with pits), oranges, grapefruit, and pears all have relatively low G.I. values. Tropical fruits like bananas, mangoes, and papayas tend to be a bit higher. Sadly, melons are typically higher on the index (Brand-Miller et al., *The Glucose Revolution*). Berries (blueberries, strawberries, boysenberries, blackberries) are all good choices because their fiber content is high.

Fat

Foods high in fat have a lower glycemic value, apparently because fat slows down the rate at which the stomach empties. This, in turn, affects the rate at which food is digested in the lower intestine. Be aware, however, that this does not mean that fatty foods are the key to low glycemic eating. French fries, because of their fat content, have a lower glycemic value than mashed potatoes; however, you don't want to make a practice of snacking on oily French fries—the fat content presents a whole other host of dietary problems. Although some diets, most notably the Atkins diet, cause their users to shed weight by reducing carbohydrate intake and replacing it with unlimited amounts of meat and fat, we do not advocate a high fat content in your diet because of its link to heart disease and other medical problems. It is possible to lose weight on a balanced eating plan without resorting to diets that cause you to lose weight by going to extremes, which causes imbalances in other regards.

The list in table 1.1 is a brief overview of the glycemic index. Remember that several factors affect glycemic index values. While a number may appear high here, it will create a lesser response in blood glucose levels if consumed with other low glycemic foods and/or with factors affecting the index, such as fat or acid content.

TABLE 1.1

Glycemic Index Values

Food Description	Amounts	G.I. Factor
Breads		
Bagel	1 small, plain, 2.3 oz	72
Dark rye, black bread	1 slice, 1.7 oz	76
French baguette	1 oz	95
Hamburger bun, prepackaged	1.5 oz	61
Pumpernickel, whole grain	1 slice, 1 oz	51
Rye bread	1 slice, 1 oz	65
Sourdough	1 slice, 1.5 oz	52
White	1 slice, 1 oz	70 (av)
100% stoneground wheat	1 slice, 1.5 oz	53
Whole wheat	1 slice, 1 oz	69 (av)
Cereals		
All-Bran with extra fiber, Kellogg's	½ cup, 1 oz	51 (av)
Cheerios, General Mills	1 cup, 1 oz	74
Grape-Nuts, Post	¼ cup, 1 oz	67
Oatmeal, old fashioned, cooked	½ cup	49

Food Description	Amounts	G.I. Factor
Shredded Wheat, Post	1 oz	67
Special K, Kellogg's	1 cup, 1 oz	54

Crackers

Food Description	Amounts	G.I. Factor
Graham crackers	4 squares, 1 oz	74
Stoned wheat thins	3 crackers, ⅖ oz	67

Dairy

Food Description	Amounts	G.I. Factor
Ice cream, 10% fat, vanilla	½ cup	61 (av)
Ice milk, vanilla	½ cup	50
Milk, skim	1 cup, 8 oz	32
Soy milk	1 cup, 8 oz	31
Yogurt, nonfat, plain	8 oz	14
Yogurt, nonfat, fruit flavored, artificial sweetener	8 oz	14

Fruit

Food Description	Amounts	G.I. Factor
Apple	1 med.	38 (av)
Banana, raw	1 med., 5 oz	55 (av)
Cherries	10 large, 3 oz	22
Dates, dried	5, 1.4 oz	103
Grapes, green	1 cup, 3 oz	46 (av)
Orange, navel	1 med., 4 oz	44 (av)
Orange juice	1 cup, 8 oz	58 (av)
Pear, fresh	1 med., 5 oz	38 (av)
Pineapple, fresh	2 slices, 4 oz	66
Watermelon	1 cup, 5 oz	72

Grains

Food Description	Amounts	G.I. Factor
Basmati rice, white, boiled	1 cup, 6 oz	58
Brown rice	1 cup, 6 oz	55 (av)

Food Description	Amounts	G.I. Factor
Bulgur, cooked	½ cup, 3 oz	48 (av)
Short grain, white	1 cup, 6 oz	72

Starches

Beans, Lentils, Pasta, Starchy Vegetables

Corn, sweet, canned, drained	½ cup	55 (av)
Lentils, green and brown, boiled	½ cup, 3 oz	30 (av)
Lentils, red, boiled	1.4 cups	26
Lima beans, baby, frozen	½ cup	32
Linguini, thick	1 cup, 6 oz	46 (av)
Macaroni, cooked	1 cup, 6 oz	45
Pinto beans, canned	½ cup	45
Spaghetti, whole wheat, cooked	1 cup	37 (av)

Potatoes

Mashed, instant	½ cup, 3.5 oz	86
New, unpeeled, boiled	5 small	62
Sweet, peeled, boiled	½ cup, 3 oz	54
White skin, with skin, baked	1 med., 4 oz	85 (av)

Miscellaneous

Angel food cake	½ cake, 1 oz	67
Banana bread	1 slice, 3 oz	47
Blueberry muffin	1 muffin, 2 oz	59
Chocolate, bar	1.5 oz	49
Peanuts, roasted, salted	½ cup	14 (av)
Sponge cake, plain	1 slice, 3.5 oz	46

Food Description	Amounts	G.I. Factor
Sugars		
Fructose, pure	3 pkt	23 (av)
Glucose, powder	2½ tabs	102
Honey	1 tbsp	58
Maltose (maltodextrin), pure	10 g	105
Sucrose	1 tsp	65 (av)

Reproduced with permission from *The Glucose Revolution: The Authoritative Guide to the Glycemic Index* (New York: Marlowe & Company, 1999).

To recap what we've said in this section about the glycemic index, here are a few important points to remember.

* Low glycemic foods are preferable to high glycemic foods.
* You should not assume the glycemic value of a certain food; the value is affected by many factors. Eating foods in combination also impacts the total glycemic value. The level at which a food raises your blood sugar level can only be accurately ascertained through testing; therefore, you should refer to a glycemic index for true values, such as the one that can be found in *The Glucose Revolution: The Authoritative Guide to the Glycemic Index*, (Brand-Miller et al.).
* The method of cooking and preparation affects the glycemic value of a food, because it impacts the physical state of starch. Cooked starch becomes gelatinized, increasing the rate of digestion and raising the glycemic value. Combinations of foods also determine the total glycemic index value of foods.
* Fiber and/or acid content will beneficially lower a food's glycemic value because they slow the rate of digestion. Try to introduce fiber into your diet with foods such as vegetables, fruits, and whole grains. Acid can be introduced into the diet by using vinegar and/or lemon as a salad dressing or marinade.

* Fat content can give a food a lower glycemic value because fat slows down gastric emptying; however, we do not recommend eating fatty foods in excess because of their association with heart disease and other medical problems.

The USDA Food Guide Pyramid

The Food Guide Pyramid was established by the United States Department of Agriculture (USDA) to provide the general public with a tool used to maintain a sound, nutritionally sufficient diet. In our modern, fast-paced world, where many people grab quick but fat-laden meals at fast food restaurants and consume inordinate amounts of sugar, the necessity for such a tool is evident.

We explain the pyramid in order to broaden the number of tools we place at your disposal to help you make educated dietary choices; however, we are not making any dietary suggestions. In order to determine your specific nutritional needs, you should further consult your doctor, diabetes educator, or dietitian.

Figure 1.1 is the USDA's Food Guide Pyramid for general adult and teen populations. Recently, the USDA established a Food Guide Pyramid for young children. Special populations have specific pyramids, as well. The American Diabetic Association (ADA) has revised the pyramid to meet the needs of people with diabetes.

The pyramid emphasizes five food groups and also includes a group for foods that are not nutritionally dense, like sugar. The tip of the pyramid is for the group that should be consumed the *least* (hence, it is the smallest). There are no specific recommendations for this group, which contains fats, oils, and sweets. These items should be consumed sparingly. As you progress down the pyramid, the food groups contain nutrient-dense foods that are recommended in order to fulfill your daily needs for vitamins, minerals, and fiber.

On the second level of the pyramid, you will see the milk, yogurt, and cheese group, as well as the meat, poultry, fish, dry beans, eggs, and

FIGURE I.I

The U.S. Department of Agriculture and the U.S. Department of Health and Human Services Food Guide Pyramid

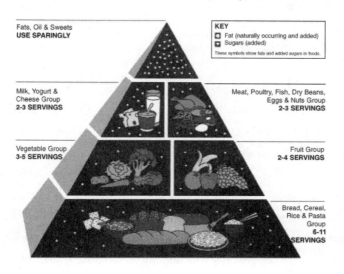

nuts group. It is recommended that you consume two to three servings per day from the milk, yogurt, and cheese group, and two to three servings per day from the meat, poultry, fish, dry beans, eggs, and nuts group. This will ensure that you receive adequate levels of calcium, protein, zinc, and iron.

On the third level, the vegetable and fruit groups are found. It is recommended that you consume three to five servings from the vegetable group and two to four servings from the fruit group. Finally, the base of the Pyramid recommends the foods that should be consumed the most. This group is the bread, cereal, rice, and pasta group, for which six to eleven servings are recommended per day. These groups contain vitamins and minerals, as well as fiber, which is critical to your digestion.

To recap, the following are the amounts of servings per food group per day that you should consume.

* Fats, oils, and sweets   sparingly
* Milk, yogurt, and cheese   2–3 servings

* Meat, poultry, fish, dry beans, eggs, and nuts   2–3 servings
* Vegetables   3–5 servings
* Fruit   2–4 servings
* Bread, cereal, rice, and pasta   6–11 servings

The triangles and squares in the tip of the pyramid represent sugar and fat, respectively. You'll notice that these symbols are also found in various groups; one example is the group at the base of the pyramid. While it is recommended that you consume grains, some are high in both fat and sugar. While a serving of whole grain bread is healthy, a butter croissant—which is refined and full of fat—is not. Again, you should make yourself aware of various foods and their respective amounts of fat and sugar. The food composition tables in the Appendix provide the appropriate information you'll need to make these choices.

So what constitutes a food serving? We've provided the various foods from the exchange list; the serving sizes are the same. Some examples are:

* Milk, yogurt, and cheese   1 cup milk, 1 cup yogurt, 1–1½ oz cheese
* Meat, etc.   3 oz chicken, 1 egg (1 oz), 1 oz nuts
* Vegetable   ½ cup cooked or raw broccoli (as an example)
* Fruit   1 small to medium apple, ½ cup fruit salad
* Bread, etc.   1 slice bread, ½ cup pasta, ½ bagel

With the glycemic index in mind, we suggest that you choose whole, unrefined foods whenever possible. There is no question that whole grain bread is more nutritious than a muffin or croissant that has been made from refined grains. We should also note that there are several camps that believe in the benefits of restricting carbohydrates, especially for weight loss. It is up to you, in conjunction with your physician or dietitian, to determine what works best for you. Your emphasis should always be on two essential things: keeping your blood sugars in control and maintaining a nutritionally sound program that provides all the essential nutrients.

When tailoring the pyramid to meet the specific needs of people with diabetes, the ADA has made a few important changes. Listed below are the significant alterations.

* Cheese is included in the Meat, poultry, etc. group.
* Beans are included in the Bread, cereal, etc. group. While beans are very high in protein, they contain as much carbohydrate as a slice of bread. Beans are fiber dense and make a great food, because they seem to make your blood sugars rise more slowly. Half of a cup constitutes one serving.
* Alcohol is included in the Fats, oils, and sweets group. Again, alcohol is nonnutritive and one drink should be counted, if consumed, as two servings of fat (one serving provides 45 calories).

Exchange Lists

Exchange lists have long been a method used for diabetic meal planning. There are six categories in the exchange lists.

1. Starch/bread
2. Fruit
3. Milk/dairy
4. Meat
5. Vegetables
6. Fat

These groupings are based on similarities in nutrient content. Each category is given a specific amount of carbohydrate, fat, and protein (although, in reality, there may be small variations in nutrient content).

We've provided these lists for two reasons. First, many publications, including diabetic cookbooks, often utilize the exchange list information. Second, the exchange list provides an easy and accurate method of counting carbohydrates, which has become even more popular with the boon of low carbohydrate diets.

Table 1.2 provides a quick glance at the exchange lists. Each grouping of foods is followed by an *average* gram and *average* calorie amount.

TABLE 1.2

Exchange List

Per serving	Carbohydrate (g)	Protein (g)	Fat (g)	Calories
Starch/bread	15	3	trace	80
Fruit	15	0	0	60
Milk/dairy				
skim	12	8	trace	90
low fat	12	8	5	120
whole	12	8	8	150
Meat				
lean	0	7	3	55
medium fat	0	7	5	75
high fat	0	7	8	100
Vegetable	5	2	0	25
Fat	0	0	5	45

Tables 1.3 through 1.8 provide serving sizes of foods from each category. Again, this is one of many tools to utilize while planning your diabetic meals. By recognizing portion sizes alone, you will get a sense

of how many carbohydrates you are consuming. There are other variables, of course, such as the amount of fat used in food preparation. This is a helpful, quick method to assess your dietary intake.

TABLE 1.3

Starch/Bread List

Per serving: Carbohydrate 15 g	Protein 3 g	Fat trace	Calories 80

Food Item	Serving Size
Bagel	½ (1 oz)
Beans	½ cup
Bread, rye	1 slice (1 oz)
Bread, white	1 slice (1 oz)
Bread, whole wheat	1 slice (1 oz)
Bulgur, cooked	½ cup
Corn	½ cup
Corn, on the cob	1 (6 in.)
Cream of Wheat, cooked	½ cup
English muffin	½ (1 oz)
Graham crackers	3 squares
Hamburger bun	½ (1 oz)
Lentils, cooked	⅓ cup
Matzoh	¾ oz
Oatmeal, cooked	½ cup
Pasta, cooked	½ cup
Peas, green	½ cup
Popcorn, air popped, no fat	3 cups
Potato, baked	1 small (3 oz)
Potato, mashed	½ cup
Pretzels	¾ oz
Rice, white or brown, cooked	⅓ cup

Shredded Wheat	½ cup
Squash, winter	1 cup
Tortilla	1 (6 in.)
Whole wheat crackers, no fat added	2–4 pieces
Yam, sweet potato, plain	⅓ cup

TABLE I.4

Fruit List

Per Serving: Carbohydrate 15 g	Protein 0 g	Fat 0 g	Calories 60
Food Item		**Serving Size**	
Apple		1 small	
Apple juice		½ cup	
Applesauce		½ cup	
Apricots, dried		7 halves	
Apricots, raw		4 small	
Banana		1 small, ½ med.	
Blueberries, raw		¾ cup	
Cantaloupe, cubed		1 cup	
Cherries		12	
Fruit cocktail, unsweetened		½ cup	
Grapefruit		½ med.	
Grapes		15	
Kiwi		1 large	
Mango		½ med.	
Nectarine		1 small	
Orange		1 small	
Orange juice		½ cup	
Papaya		1 cup	
Peach		1 med.	

Pear	1 small
Pineapple, fresh	¾ cup
Plum	2 small
Prunes	3 med.
Raisins	2 tbsp
Raspberries	1 cup
Strawberries, raw	1¼ cups
Watermelon, cubed	1¼ cups

TABLE 1.5

Milk/Dairy List

Skim

Per Serving:

Carbohydrate 12 g	Protein 8 g	Fat trace	Calories 90

Food Item	Serving Size
Dry nonfat milk	⅓ cup
Low fat buttermilk	1 cup
1% milk	1 cup
Plain nonfat yogurt	8 oz
Skim milk	1 cup

Low fat

Per Serving:

Carbohydrate 12 g	Protein 8 g	Fat 5 g	Calories 120

Food Item	Serving Size
Evaporated whole milk	½ cup
Plain low fat yogurt	8 oz

Whole

Per Serving: Carbohydrate 12 g	Protein 8 g	Fat 8 g	Calories 150

Food Item	Serving Size
Plain whole yogurt	8 oz
2% milk	1 cup
Whole milk	1 cup

TABLE 1.6

Meat List

Lean

Per serving: Carbohydrate 0 g	Protein 7 g	Fat 3 g	Calories 55

Food Item	Serving Size
Beef, flank	1 oz
Beef, round	1 oz
Beef, sirloin	1 oz
Beef, tenderloin	1 oz
Cheese, cottage	¼ cup
Cheese, parmesan	2 tbsp
Chicken, without skin	1 oz
Cornish hen, without skin	1 oz
Egg whites	3
Egg, substitute	½ cup
Fish, fresh, all types	1 oz
Fish, frozen, all types	1 oz
Game (pheasant, rabbit, venison), no skin	1 oz
Herring, uncreamed, smoked	1 oz
Luncheon meats, 95% fat free	1½ oz
Pork, lean (ham, tenderloin)	1 oz

Food Item	Serving Size
Sardines, canned	2 med.
Shellfish (crab, lobster, shrimp, scallops), fresh	2 oz
Tuna, water packed	1 oz
Veal, chop, roasts	1 oz

Medium fat

Per serving:

Carbohydrate 0 g	Protein 7 g	Fat 5 g	Calories 75

Food Item	Serving Size
Beef, ground	1 oz
Beef, roast	1 oz
Beef, steak (porterhouse, T-bone)	1 oz
Cheese, skim or part skim, ricotta	1 oz
Chicken, with skin	1 oz
Duck	1 oz
Egg	1
Lamb	1 oz
Organ meats (liver, kidney)	1 oz
Pork, chops, loin	1 oz
Salmon, canned	1 oz
Tofu	4 oz
Turkey, ground	1 oz
Veal, cutlet	1 oz

High fat

Per serving:

Carbohydrate 0 g	Protein 7 g	Fat 8 g	Calories 100

Food Item	Serving Size
Beef, USDA Prime, ribs	1 oz
Cheese, cheddar, Swiss, Monterey Jack	1 oz

Frankfurter, chicken or turkey	1
Luncheon meat, bologna, salami	1 oz
Peanut butter	1 tbsp
Pork, ribs	1 oz
Sausage	1 oz

TABLE I.7

Vegetable List

Per Serving:			
Carbohydrates 5 g	Protein 2 g	Fat 0 g	Calories 25

Food Item	Serving Size
Artichoke	1 small, ½ med.
Asparagus	½ cup
Beans, green	½ cup
Bean sprouts	½ cup
Beets	½ cup
Broccoli	½ cup
Brussels sprouts	½ cup
Cabbage, cooked	½ cup
Carrots	½ cup
Cauliflower	½ cup
Eggplant	½ cup
Greens, collard	½ cup
Kohlrabi	½ cup
Leeks	½ cup
Mushrooms, cooked	½ cup
Okra	½ cup
Onions	½ cup
Peas, snap	½ cup
Peppers, red, green, yellow	½ cup
Rutabaga	½ cup
Sauerkraut	½ cup

Spinach, cooked	½ cup
Tomato	1 med.–large
Tomato juice	½ cup
Turnips	½ cup
Water chestnuts	½ cup
Zucchini, cooked	½ cup

TABLE 1.8

Fat List

Per Serving:			
Carbohydrates 0 g	Protein 0 g	Fat 5 g	Calories 45

Food Item	Serving Size
Avocado	⅛ med.
Bacon*	1 slice
Butter*	1 tsp
Cream cheese*	1 tbsp
Cream, light*	2 tbsp
Cream, heavy*	1 tbsp
Margarine	1 tsp
Mayonnaise	1 tsp
Nuts, most varieties	1 tbsp
Oil	1 tsp
Olives	10 small
Seeds, most varieties	1 tbsp

*Fats with this symbol denote saturated fats.

Note: When looking at labels, always check for fat amount. Products such as salad dressings and reduced calorie products will vary and for that reason have been omitted.

Free Food List

There are several beverages, condiments, and vegetables that contain low amounts of carbohydrate, protein, and fat. For that reason, these items are considered *free*, roughly providing less than 20 calories per serving. It is always wise to consider these foods *free in moderation*.

Beverages

Bouillon, fat free, with or without sodium

Carbonated drinks, sugar-free sodas, water

Coffee

Other sugar-free drinks, e.g., Crystal Light

Tea

Condiments

Catsup (limit to 1 tbsp)

Extracts (vanilla, almond, cherry, lemon, etc.)

Horseradish

Lemon juice

Lime juice

Mustard

Soy sauce

Taco sauce

Vinegar

Wine (limit ¼ cup *for cooking only*)

Worcestershire sauce

Seasonings and Spices

No limitations.

Sweet Substitutes

Gelatin, sugar-free

Gum, sugar-free

Sugar substitutes (aspartame, saccharin, Splenda, stevia)

Whipped topping (limit 2 tbsp), e.g., Cool Whip

Vegetables

Cabbage, raw

Celery

Cucumber

Endive

Escarole

Green onion

Hot peppers

Lettuce

Mushrooms, raw

Pickles, dill (limit 2–4)

Radishes

Spinach, raw

Zucchini, raw

Chapter Two

Grocery
Shopping

• • • • • • • • • • •

Sometimes the hardest part of a diet for diabetes is knowing what foods to buy. This section addresses how to navigate your grocery store, how to select healthy foods, and how to read labels. We designed these guidelines to help you seek out foods that are low in glycemic value and low in fat. Since low glycemic foods generally fall into several categories, such as fruit and vegetables, dairy products, and grains, you can create a mental map of your grocery store that speeds up the shopping process while steering clear of potential pitfalls (frozen entrées, baked goods, etc.). Within each shopping section, you need to be aware of what selections are high in fat and should be avoided.

Rule One: Stick to the Outside Aisles

Grocery stores are generally laid out with certain items in the outside aisles that are safe for people with diabetes:

fresh produce (fruits and vegetables), dairy products, meats, and grains. Highly refined foods (such as crackers, cookies, cereals, and frozen entrées) are usually found on the inside aisles. This is not to say that you can't venture in! Prepare yourself in advance by familiarizing yourself with the "safe" foods. Review the section on the glycemic index in Chapter I. Select products that are lower on the glycemic index, such as brown rice and lentils. Of course, herbs and spices are found in the inside aisles, and—since these are low glycemic—there is nothing better than a little spice to improve your culinary experience.

Rule Two: Purchase Proteins That Are Lower in Fat

Choose chicken or turkey over high fat meats such as beef and pork. Your best bet, naturally, is to load up on skinless, boneless white chicken and turkey breasts. White meat contains fewer calories than its dark meat counterpart.

Poultry with its skin on is much fattier than poultry without its skin. If you are being cost-conscious, it might be less expensive to purchase chicken breasts on the bone with its skin; just be sure to remove the skin before cooking. Ground turkey is an excellent substitute in many recipes that call for ground beef; for example, you can put ground turkey into your chili, make ground turkey burgers, or cook a ground turkey meatloaf. We've provided recipes in the recipe section for all of these healthy alternatives. Turkey needs to be more heavily spiced than beef to make it flavorful, but your taste buds will guide you.

Be aware of how certain meats are advertised. Sausage, for example, may be labeled as low fat or 97 percent fat free. These can be marketing traps, and will be explained in Rule Four. Any sausage—even turkey—tends to be high in fat, and hard on the arteries. Chicken can be a good substitute for beef or pork in Mexican entrées, like tacos and enchiladas; gumbo; soups; and any other dish you choose. Look for our chicken recipes in the recipe section, and be creative in using it to replace high fat meats in your favorite recipes.

When it does come to ordering beef and pork, loin or round cuts and select cuts usually have the lowest fat content. Prime cuts are highest in fat, because of the marbling in the meat that categorizes it as a prime cut.

Fresh seafood is usually found either in close proximity or in the same case as the meats. Depending on its preparation (that is, as long as it isn't fried), seafood is a healthy alternative to meat. Generally, fish is a very low calorie option for protein. A typical 4-ounce portion of fish (cod, halibut, sole) is roughly 130 calories. The exceptions are higher fat fishes such as mackerel and salmon. However, fat found in fish, such as omega-3 fatty acids, are nutritionally valuable fats and have been recommended as an important part of a healthy diet. In fact, omega-3 fatty acids (eicosapentaenoic acid, or EPA, and docosahexaenoic acid, or DHA) are known to act as an anticoagulant in the blood and have been associated with reducing cholesterol levels. Fish, like turkey and chicken, can be substituted in recipes that generally call for meat, such as in tacos, enchiladas, and other Mexican foods. For more caloric information on fish, refer to the food composition tables at the back of the book or any recommended calorie counter.

Rule Three: Steer Clear of Frozen Food Fiascos

Frozen food labels can be misleading. Items are packaged with claims such as "lite" and "reduced calorie," which can be very confusing for the consumer. On closer look, you will often find that these foods are laden with sodium and sugars. Avoid purchasing premade entrées if at all possible. Of course, there are some entrées that are healthy and do contain low sodium and low fat foods. But in order to be certain, you must scrutinize the labels. See pages 39–42 for details on label reading and on how to interpret this often complex information.

Look for frozen vegetables in convenient packages that are frozen fresh (in other words, no added sauces). This is an easy way to add vegetables to your diet. Simply add a bag of your favorite frozen vegetables to a soup or casserole. Throw vegetables in a pan with chicken and your favorite spices for an instant stir-fry. Frozen fruit is best when it doesn't have added sugar. Frozen berries are great for adding to your favorite smoothie or for tossing into a quick fruit salad.

Putting It Together

Consider three well-known dietetic frozen food entrées; Healthy Choice, Weight Watcher's Smart Ones, and Stouffer's Lean Cuisine. Calories are usually restricted to less than 300 calories per serving (the amount in one package). Ingredients vary widely due to the type of entrée purchased. Because of shelf life concerns, many products contain high sodium levels, averaging 700 milligrams per serving. Carbohydrate amounts also vary according to the specific entrées. Both Healthy Choice and Smart Ones provide exchange list values. Healthy Choice has the lowest sodium content.

Compare Stouffer's Lean Cuisine Hearty Portions Meal Grilled Chicken and Penne Pasta to Stouffer's regular Penne Pasta and Chicken Bake, as follows:

* Lean Cuisine Hearty Portions Meal (14 oz)
  360 calories   47 g carbohydrate   7 g fat   870 mg sodium

* Stouffer's (11.5 oz)
  340 calories   37 g carbohydrate   14 g fat   1,040 mg sodium

At first glance, it may appear that the Stouffer's regular is a good choice because it contains fewer calories and carbohydrates than the lean variety—but look again. After recalculating the 14-ounce Lean Cuisine Hearty Portions to equal the Stouffer's regular 11.5-ounce serving, the lean variety contains 296 calories, 39 grams of carbohydrate, 6 grams of fat, and 714 milligrams of sodium. Remember to look at your labels carefully when choosing frozen foods, and always take into consideration the variations in serving sizes.

Rule Four: Watch Out for Traps in Marketing

When you do your shopping, take time to assess which foods provide your body with the nutrients it needs. You probably know that it is important to watch out for highly refined carbohydrate-type foods and foods high in fat, just as you also pay special attention to labels—but do you really know what you're getting?

Keep in mind that food companies are very adept at promoting their products with catchy phrases and seductive packaging. Be especially aware of the key words often used to entice the unwary buyer.

Lite

Lite or *light* doesn't mean low fat or low sugar. While it may be used to indicate this, it might also be referring merely to the consistency of the product. *Light* cheesecake may contain just as much fat and sugar, only with more whipped texture. An olive oil might be lighter in color, but contain just as much fat. *Light* might also be used to denote fewer calories than the *original* product, but not necessarily fewer calories in general. Always check the labels, especially when a manufacturer may be employing this common marketing gimmick.

Sugar Free

This term often means *sucrose* free, or free of table sugar. Other sugars you should look for include maltose (maltodextrin), fructose, corn syrup, and honey.

This ploy can be seen in many diabetic cookies. Often, these are sweetened with fructose, which is known to create a slow rise in blood sugar levels, but fructose is still a form of sugar. In other words, the carbohydrate content is no less than those foods made with sucrose (for those of you counting carbohydrates), and the amount of calories is no less as well. Honey is often billed as the *natural sweetener*. Be careful of this trick, too. It is just as potent as table sugar and contains just as many calories. If you recall, maltose is two glucose molecules, and will rapidly raise blood sugar levels.

Cholesterol Free

All vegetable fats are cholesterol free. Don't confuse *cholesterol free* with *healthy fats*. Often, vegetable oils (which are inherently cholesterol free) are hydrogenated (made solid), which renders these fats partially saturated. A cracker might boast that it is cholesterol free. This means there are no animal fats (such as lard) used in the processing. This doesn't mean it is a healthy choice. It could still be high in saturated fats, such as the hydrogenated vegetable oils used in manufacturing.

"Fill in Blank Here" Percent Fat-Free

Be careful with this claim. If a product claims to be a certain percentage fat-free, it is referring to the product's total weight; it is not referring to the percentage of fat calories per serving. For example, the producer of a luncheon meat might claim that it is 95 percent fat-free (compared to an original product). This means that the total weight (in grams) of the package is 5 percent fat. This does not mean that per serving, the luncheon meat has 5 percent of calories from fat; it might be as high as 45 percent. Check the label reading section of this chapter for instructions on calculating fat calories.

Dietetic

Be especially careful with this label. It means that one or more ingredients have been altered in some fashion, such as restricted or substituted. This does not refer to a reduction in calories. For example, look at a "dietetic" salad dressing. In order to reduce fat, manufacturers will often increase sugar. This creates a better mouth feel (by adding starches for consistency) and improves the taste. However, the calories are often the same as in nondietetic products. The same is often true for other "dietetic" items, such as cookies and crackers.

Sugar Substitutes

Labeling laws allow food companies to claim that a product contains *0 grams* of any nutrient if it is under 0.5 grams per serving. Foods that contain sugar substitutes often have *0 grams* listed under total carbohydrates (refer to the label reading section of this chapter). This, too, can be misleading. The following is a list of several sugar substitutes often used:

* Aspartame—commonly known as NutraSweet or Equal
* Saccharine—commonly known as Sweet'N Low or Sugar Twin
* Acesulfame-K—commonly known as Sweet One
* Sucralose—commonly known as Splenda (also contains maltodextrin and dextrose)
* Xylitol—sugar alcohol
* Maltitol—sugar alcohol
* Sorbitol—sugar alcohol
* Stevia—natural herb that is several times sweeter than sugar

While some medical experts claim that sugar substitutes (particularly sugar alcohols) have little impact on blood sugar levels, we think it is prudent to be aware of these substitutes, and use your own discretion in choosing whether or not to consume them. In fact, there are some researchers that believe that nonnutritive sugar substitutes such as aspartame do create an insulinemic response.

Drs. Richard and Rachael Heller, famed authors of the popular book *The Carbohydrate Addict's Healthy Heart Program*, suggest that sugar substitutes cause a rapid rise in insulin because the body handles the substitute sweetener as if it were *real* sugar—signaling a response to the body to release insulin. The result is an elevated level of insulin which leads to fat storage. Will blood sugar levels be increased? Probably not, but the elevated level of insulin signals fat storage and increased appetite.

Another word about the sweetener controversy. Many of you have read propaganda over the Internet suggesting that nonnutritive sweeteners have negative side effects, such as aspartame leading to symptoms of multiple sclerosis, lupus, and other such illnesses. One rumor even suggests that the artificial sweeteners produce formaldehyde in the body!

Some people may indeed have sensitivities to sweeteners, but the majority of this information is alarmist. People with sensitivities to sweeteners may report minor side effects such as gastric distress (loose stools, gas, bloating) with the use of sugar alcohols, but no more so than the incidence of side effects with the use of virtually any product. Use your own discretion when using sweeteners and weigh the pros and cons individually.

Putting It Together

We purchased three varieties of vanilla ice cream from the same manufacturer: One was regular, one was "no sugar added," and the last was "light." See table 2.1 for the comparisons.

TABLE 2.1

Comparisons of Vanilla Ice Cream

Amount	Calories per serving	Fat grams per serving	Carbohydrate grams per serving
Regular			
½ cup	160	10	15
No Sugar Added			
½ cup	90	4.5	11
Light			
½ cup	130	4.5	18

The "regular" variety was made with some basic ingredients such as milk, cream, sugar, and egg yolks (in that order). The "no sugar added" also listed sugar alcohols on the label and has maltodextrin (another name for maltose, which is two glucose molecules) as an ingredient. The "light" version has sugar listed as the second ingredient and corn syrup as the third ingredient. Clearly, "light" refers to reduced fat as compared to the *regular product*. It actually contains more sugar and total carbohydrates (which includes sugar) than the regular ice cream! The better choice would be the "no sugar added" variety, but be conscientious of maltodextrin as an ingredient. The lesson here is simple: Read labels carefully before grabbing a package that appears to be safe, and stick to the serving size!

Let's Go Shopping

Now that we've told you what to watch out for, here are some guidelines to help make your grocery shopping easy, healthy, and productive.

Fresh Produce

It is wise to begin in the fresh produce section when you shop as this is the area where you should stockpile. Load up on fresh vegetables and fruits. Remember, your objective is to consume two to four fruits a day and three to five vegetables a day (according to the Food Guide Pyramid). Keeping this—as well as low glycemic choices—in mind, create a list for one week's worth of shopping.

Our Recommendations
Fruit
You will want to purchase at least fourteen pieces of fruit for each person per week. This meets the minimum requirement for fruits according to the Food Guide Pyramid (two servings a day). Choose whole fruits, since dried fruits can be very high in sugar (for example, dates

have a higher glycemic index value than glucose powder). Apples, pears, and plums are among our favorites; they have low glycemic values and are easy to pack to take with you! Each person with diabetes has a sense of which fruits do not suit him. Learn which fruits are most easily tolerated by you, and stock up on these. Bring them to your place of work and keep them readily available to you at all times in case of emergency. Berries are also great choices; you can add them to cereal, cottage cheese, and salads. They're also great for snacking. Grocery stores now carry an assortment of precut fruits for salads and other uses. If preparation and convenience are an issue, think about purchasing these items to save yourself some preparation time.

Potatoes

Stock up on yams, sweet potatoes, and new potatoes. To store potatoes, place them in a paper bag (do not store in plastic), and keep them in a cool, dark place. Potatoes were originally stored in cellars . . . think of cellar climates when finding a place in your home.

Vegetables

For vegetables, there are no limits. Always keep fixings on hand for salads, such as lettuce, cucumbers, tomatoes, and peppers. If convenience is an issue, purchase precut, prewashed packages of lettuce and vegetables. Grocery stores often carry premade salads in an assortment of choices such as Greek and Caesar salads. Add your own low sugar, low fat dressing and you have a convenient accompaniment to any meal.

Special Cuts of Protein Foods

Remember your option of requesting special cuts at the meat, poultry, and seafood counters. For example, ask your butcher to remove all visible fats from any cuts of meat. As we've said, the higher grade cut you choose, the higher the fat content (marbling). Choose leaner cuts of beef. Some additional tips follow:

* Have your butcher prewrap individual serving sizes in the amount to be consumed. For example, if ordering fish, have your butcher wrap individual fillets of 4 to 5 ounces each. This helps with portion control, and saves you time and effort.
* Have the dates of purchase on packages of any meat, fish, and poultry. While beef can stay in the freezer for longer periods of time, fish does not keep well beyond three months.
* Purchase large packs of chicken. Individually wrap the chicken and freeze it for storage. Often, larger packs of chicken are less expensive.

Dairy

Some people tolerate dairy products better than others. Hidden sugars can be found in a variety of dairy products, so pay close attention to the labels.

* Yogurt, while healthy, may be full of sugar. Choose nonfat varieties sweetened with artificial sweetener. Some fruit-sweetened yogurts contain as much as 45 grams of carbohydrate per serving! Those sweetened with artificial sweetener have a *very* low glycemic index value.
* Nonfat cottage cheese is an excellent source of calcium and protein. This can also be purchased in individual serving size containers.
* Nonfat milk is an essential. In a pinch, when you need a snack, milk has a great balance of protein and carbohydrate. It has a low glycemic value, as well.

Breads

Bakeries can be difficult to navigate as there are so many varieties that it can be overwhelming to choose properly. Here are some helpful hints:

* Remember to check for fiber grams. Your daily goals for fiber intake, on average, should be *30 to 35 grams.* This is the best place to start. Breads such as Orowheat Light offer 4 grams of fiber per serving!

* Avoid white, refined breads. Sourdough is an exception, since the glycemic value tends to be low due to the acid content in the bread.

* Stick to *whole* grains. Wheat bread can be as nutritionally void as refined bread. Remember—you want fiber.

* Beware of hidden fats. Croissants, muffins, and bakery breads such as banana bread are all laden with dietary fats.

* Serving size alert! Deli-size bagels are not typical servings. One bagel can pack a walloping 60 grams of carbohydrate.

* Avoid items such as coffee cakes, doughnuts, and other assorted pastries. These are loaded with fat, sugar, and refined flour.

Cereals

Have you ever been completely overwhelmed in the cereal section of your supermarket? There are so many varieties, and it seems that every day a new product emerges . . . usually some variation on your child's favorite candy bar. It doesn't take a whole lot of energy to determine that these are perhaps not the wisest choices, but—beyond the obvious—what do you choose?

* Choose the old-fashioned kind of cereal; oats are far superior to any processed cereal. Oats have a high fiber content and contain a reasonable amount of carbohydrate per serving. Of course, don't sweeten your cereal with sugar.

* Bran cereals, such as All Bran or oat bran, also contain a great deal of fiber and seem to have relatively low glycemic index values.

* Be wary of cereals with added fruit. These often pack a great

deal of carbohydrate. Remember that dried fruit, such as dates, can have extremely high glycemic index values.

* Cereals claiming to have low sugar contents do not exclude sugars having high glycemic index values.

Grains, Beans, and Pasta

These foods can be kept in storage for long periods of time. The key is to store them in airtight containers. These foods provide a variety of nutrients and fiber, and are recommended for a heart-healthy diet. For people with diabetes, the amount is always a consideration. For some, these types of foods might be restricted. Again, seek out the help of a professional to determine what is appropriate for you. To help you make the wisest choices (you determine the quantities you may consume), here are a few recommended staples for your household.

* Brown rice is great for casseroles, with stir-fries, or in soups. It has a low glycemic index value.
* Beans and lentils are high in fiber and have low glycemic values. These are great for soups, chili, and in salads. Rinse canned beans thoroughly to rid them of excess salt.
* Bulgur and barley are nice alternatives to ordinary rice.
* Pasta; choose whole wheat. Some data shows that different varieties of pasta are lower in glycemic value, such as fettuccine. We suggest that you test your blood sugar to see how it affects you. Use pasta as an accompaniment to dinner, not as a main dish.

Spices, Dressings, and Other Miscellaneous Items

Condiments can be tricky. They are often high in sugar and fat, and can pose the biggest threat to a healthy shopping excursion.

* Herbs and spices are safe choices when stocking your cupboard with staples. There is no better way to dress up any meal than by adding a mélange of flavor, and these are indispensa-

ble. Keep your cupboard full of the following: garlic powder, pepper, basil, tarragon, lemon pepper, sage, oregano, curry, chili powder, dry mustard, marjoram, cinnamon, nutmeg, and other dried spices such as Chinese five spice. Always keep on hand a sugar substitute and a butter substitute, such as Butter Buds, in the cupboard. I Can't Believe It's Not Butter! Spray works well on vegetables.

* Keep the following in supply at all times: Dijon mustard, olive oil, low-sodium soy sauce, balsamic vinegar, and white wine vinegar. You never know when you'll need to whip up a quick dressing or marinade.

* Choose salad dressings that are low in sugar and fat. Some suggested brand names are Rising Sun Farm and Follow Your Heart.

* *Stock* up! Keep chicken, beef, and vegetable stock available either in granule or canned form. *Stocks can be used to substitute for fat in cooking, cup for cup.* Don't be caught without backup stock; it's an easy and healthy way to add flavor to recipes. Granules are easy to keep in storage for long periods of time. Be sure to store them in a dry area.

Label Reading

Nutrition labels provide you with a great deal of information; however, all of that information can be very confusing if you don't know how to interpret it. We'll help you master the art of reading nutrition labels with the label from a can of beans as an example (see table 2.2).

TABLE 2.2

Sample Label

Nutrition Facts

Serving Size ½ cup (133g)

Servings Per Container 3 **(A)**

Calories 100 **(B)**

Calories from Fat 0 **(C)**

Amount Per Serving	**% Daily Value***	
Total Fat 0g	0%	
Saturated Fat 0g	0%	
Cholesterol 0 mg	0%	
Sodium 300 mg	15%	
Total Carbohydrate 18g	6%	**(D)**
Dietary Fiber 5g	20%	**(E)**
Sugars less than 1g		
Protein 7g		

Vitamin A 0% • Vitamin C 2% • Calcium 2% • Iron 10%   **(F)**

*Percent Daily Values are based on a 2,000 calorie diet. (Your daily values may be higher or lower depending on your calorie needs.)

	Calories:	2,000	2,500	
Total Fat	Less than	65g	80g	
Saturated Fat	Less than	20g	25g	
Cholesterol	Less than	300mg	300mg	
Sodium	Less than	2,400mg	2,400mg	**(G)**
Total Carbohydrate		300g	375g	
Dietary Fiber		25g	30g	

Calories Per Gram:

Fat 9   Carbohydrate 4   Protein 4

INGREDIENTS: BEANS, WATER, SALT. **(H)**

(A) Serving size is specifically noted; this is important! A serving size is not the entire can. When calculating your daily intake of carbohydrates—regardless of which method you choose to use—be aware of how many servings you're consuming.

(B) Calories represent the amount of calories *per serving*. (In this example, it provides 100 calories per ½ cup beans.)

(C) This represents the amount of calories from fat. Another way to determine the percentage of calories from fat is to multiply the fat grams by nine. For example, if the total fat is 2 grams, the calories are 18 or 9 times 2 grams. Take this number (18) and divide it by the total calories per serving (in this case, 100 calories). Eighteen divided by 100 equals 0.18, or 18 percent. This product derives 18 percent of its calories from fat.

(D) The total amount of carbohydrate is listed here. For example, out of 18 grams of carbohydrate, 5 of those grams are from fiber—a good choice! Remember that fiber is a factor in low glycemic eating. Do not add the amount of fiber and sugar to the total carbohydrate amount; this will only confuse you. When counting carbohydrates, look at the total carbohydrate amount listed in grams.

(E) The percent represented here is Percent Daily Values, which are based on a 2,000-calorie-per-day diet. This might not work for you, however. If you are on a 1,500-calorie-per-day diet, these numbers do not apply to you. In addition, do not confuse these percentages with the amount of nutrients per serving size of the product. In this example, one serving size of beans has 18 grams of carbohydrate. The product provides 72 percent of its calories from carbohydrate, not 6 percent. How do we arrive at the figure 72 percent? Eighteen grams times 4 (the number of calories per gram of carbohydrate) equals 72 calories from carbohydrate. Seventy-two divided by 100 equals 0.72, or 72 percent being calories from carbohydrate.

(F) This portion of the label provides information on micronutrients, such as vitamin and mineral content. Depending on the product and the amount of fortification (that is, adding vitamins to products), this portion of the label will vary.

(G) This portion of the label breaks down nutrient needs based on a 2,000-calorie- and a 2,500-calorie-per-day diet. Your needs may vary. Pay special attention to carbohydrate recommendations; these may be too high for your diabetic needs.

(H) The list of ingredients is in order from the greatest amount of ingredients to the least. Generally, the first three to five ingredients listed comprise the bulk of the food item.

Equipped with knowing what marketing traps to look out for, and how to read product labels, you're ready to go out and shop. Just remember that terms like *light* and *low fat* that are used to entice buyers can often be misleading, and to take into account varying serving sizes when comparing products.

Chapter Three

Eating Out in Restaurants

· · · · · · · · · · · ·

Restaurants present a variety of pitfalls for the unwary diner with diabetes. We've provided simple guidelines in this chapter so that you can easily reference what you need to avoid, depending on the type of cuisine—fine dining, casual sit-down dining, or even fast food. We've given specific guidelines for cuisines including Italian, Mexican, Chinese, French, Greek, steak, seafood, salad bars, sandwich shops, diners and delis, hamburger and chicken joints, breakfast and brunch restaurants, and rotisserie chicken.

Keep in mind, as well, the simple rules provided in chapter 4, "Special Situations," that can be applied to almost any situation: Fill your plate with salad first, reserve a quarter of your plate for protein, and avoid going back for seconds.

· · ·

Italian

Beware of . . .

- ★ Cream sauces like Alfredo
- ★ Parmigiana—breaded and fried
- ★ Scallopine
- ★ Pepperoni, sausage, prosciutto—the fat content is too high
- ★ White refined breads such as focaccia and garlic bread
- ★ Cheeses—whether in cream sauces, on pizzas, or in calzones
- ★ Quantity in pasta dishes—½ cup cooked pasta is one serving

Safer to try . . .

- ★ Marinara and marsala sauces
- ★ Wine-based sauces
- ★ Red clam sauce
- ★ Grilled fish, chicken, vegetables, Portobello mushrooms—be aware of fat used in cooking
- ★ Primavera sauces with vegetables
- ★ Pasta as a side dish
- ★ Seafood sauces—these can still be high in butter or oil (ask your server)
- ★ Minestrone

Tips . . .

- ★ Remove skin from poultry
- ★ Ask for Caesar dressing on the side and skip the croutons
- ★ Order vinaigrette on the side
- ★ Order pizza with thin crust, ½ or no cheese, and extra vegetables (some restaurants offer whole wheat crust, too, which is much better for you than crusts made with refined flour)

* Ask about cooking methods—grilled vegetables, though seemingly a safe choice, might be drenched in oil
* Choose pasta as a side dish with chicken or fish as your main dish

Ideal meal

* Grilled fish or chicken with side of vegetables and a side of pasta with marinara or primavera
* Ask that sauces (for example, marsala) be served on the side
* Ask if vegetables are prepared with butter or oil.
* Ask that vegetables be either steamed or served on the side

Mexican

Beware of . . .

* Guacamole, sour cream, cheese—all of these are very high in fat
* Refried beans (there's lard in there!)
* Flour tortilla
* Anything deep fried—that is, chips or chimichangas
* Red meats, especially ground, because the fat content is high
* Pork dishes; the fat content is high
* Corn cakes
* Rice dishes, which are often made with extra oil and spices
* Mole sauce—this is a sauce made with a chocolate base
* Quesadillas, taquitos
* Chimiflautas—beef, pork, or chicken in flour tortillas
* Carnitas
* Tamales—cornmeal used—high glycemic
* Chorizo—Mexican sausage high in fat
* Milanesa—breaded beefsteak

* Ceviche (fish, chicken, shrimp marinated in lemon-lime juice)
* Chicken tacos à la carte with corn tortillas (Beware: Some restaurants double-wrap tacos; ask for one corn tortilla only.)
* Chicken tacos in soft corn tortillas (also fish and shrimp)
* Pico de gallo instead of high fat condiments
* Enchiladas in red sauce—cheese content can still be high (ask your server)
* Whole beans, black and pinto, instead of refried beans
* Grilled chicken tostada salads, no guacamole or sour cream—and no shell (Some shells weigh in at 400 calories!)
* Use salsa and hot sauce to add flavor
* Fajitas, no oil
* Carne asada or picada—while it is beef, it is a better option than ground beef—prepared with onions
* Small bean burrito with vegetables; go light on the cheese
* Cocido—beef and vegetable soup
* Nopales—cactus; be sure to ask how it is prepared
* If ordering a burrito, opt for no cheese; try chicken instead of beef

Tips . . .

* Get spicy with hot sauces; this adds flavor without the fat
* Some restaurants use two tortillas per taco; eat one tortilla per taco (one small tortilla is considered one serving of starch)
* Ask for foods that are grilled, not deep-fried (tacos often come in fried shells)
* Ask that foods that are grilled be prepared with little oil
* Use salsa for dressing on salads
* Tortilla soup recipes vary so much from restaurant to restaurant; ask how the soup is prepared; many are clear broths with

vegetables, chicken, and some cheese; if it is thickened with masa flour or has a lot of cheese or avocado, pass

* Verde is a green sauce, Colorado is a red sauce; ask for sauces on the side

Ideal meal

* Grilled shrimp or chicken dish with whole beans as a side
* Order a dinner salad or soup if the base of the soup is broth
* Fajita dishes are fine
* Skip the rice and tortillas and eat the vegetable and meat portion only
* Tostada salads are fine, but skip the rice and beans; order with chicken omitting rice, sour cream, guacamole, and cheese, and don't eat the fried shell!

Chinese

Beware of . . .

* Sauces—these can be very high in both sugar and fat
* Deep fried items
* Fried rice and noodles
* White rice or sticky rice
* Eggrolls, potstickers, dumplings—if prepared in oil
* Duck (HIGH FAT—3 ounces has a whopping 30 grams of fat!)
* Chow mein—crispy noodles
* Lo mein—soft noodles
* Chinese chicken salad—fried noodles and high sugar dressings

Safer to try . . .

- ✶ Anything steamed, such as fish, vegetables, or chicken
- ✶ Stir-fry using water or broth
- ✶ Steamed dumplings
- ✶ Tofu dishes, both grilled and steamed; ask if a lot of oil is used in grilling
- ✶ Broth; sodium content may be high
- ✶ Brown rice
- ✶ Chinese chicken salad—order without dressing and fried noodles; ask for dressing on the side

Tips . . .

- ✶ Ask for "dry wok" method, which means boiled or steamed
- ✶ Ask about sugar content in sauces; sauces can be very high in refined sugar and starch (the stuff that creates a thick, glazed sauce)
- ✶ Opt for low-sodium soy
- ✶ If you are sensitive to MSG (monosodium glutamate), be sure to ask your server which menu selections are MSG-free

Ideal meal

- ✶ "Dry wok" stir-fried chicken or shrimp and vegetables with low-sodium soy
- ✶ If brown rice is available, ask for a side order

French

Beware of . . .

- ✶ Beurre-blanc (butter-based sauce)

* Duck
* Foie gras
* Pâté
* Sautéed dishes (high in fat)
* Escargots (made with a lot of butter)
* Pommes frites—fried shoestring potatoes
* Mousseline—these seafood molds are made with cream and mayonnaise
* Croquettes—either savory or sweet varieties are not recommended as the cooking process involves deep frying
* Filet de Boeuf en Croute—a fillet of beef encrusted in pastry

Safer to try. . .

* Bouillabaisse—various fish and shellfish in a tomato-based broth
* Fillet of sole, poached
* Scallops
* Wine-based sauces
* Haricots verts (green beans)
* Salade Niçoise

Tips. . .

* *Always* ask for sauce on the side
* Try low fat, wine-based sauces like bordelaise
* Avoid high fat sauces such as bérnaise, velouté, hollandaise, and béchamel—all are made with a *roux* as a base (a mixture of flour and butter); velouté, which is a sauce made with stock and a roux, is a base for many other sauces such as allemande, poulette, aurore, or soubise. All have small variations such as the addition of onions or tomato puree. Many sauces are also made with a brown sauce base (beef drippings and flour).

These are perigueux, lyonnaise (sauce with onions), poivrade (pepper sauce), bordelaise, and marchand de vin (wine and mushroom sauce). Restaurants may do variations on these typical French sauces (ask your server and/or chef for sauces on the side)

* Sole seems to be a favorite and there are several ways in which it is prepared. Many dishes begin with a white wine sauce and from there add whipping cream and butter. Some names to look for: veronique, duglere (a good option). Sole is a wonderfully light fish (ask for sauces on the side)

Ideal meal

* Sauces are the mainstay in French cooking; before ordering any dish, inquire about the sauce
* Ask for sole or a fillet of beef
* Begin your meal with a nice bouillabaisse or Salade Niçoise

Greek

Beware of . . .

* Moussaka—eggplant and beef casserole in cream sauce (béchamel); ask for a lighter variety if possible
* Spanakopita—spinach and cheese in filo
* Tzatziki—yogurt with cucumber and herbs (some restaurants offer low fat, as do markets—in which case, enjoy!)
* Saganaki—cheese fried in brandy
* Falafel
* Gyros

Safer to try . . .

* Avgolemono—chicken soup thickened with egg whites and lemon
* Souvlaki kabob—chicken or beef (some are marinated with a lot of oil, so ask your server)
* Grilled eggplant—ask for light on oil
* Pita—preferably whole wheat if offered; one-half a pita equals one serving of starch
* Hummus—can be high in fat, so use sparingly
* Dolmas—stuffed grape leaves; ask about the oil content, because it can run high
* Greek salad
* Roasted eggplant dip

Tips . . .

* Since Mediterranean cuisine uses a lot of oil, always ask about olive oil content in the dishes you order
* Ask for a side salad, and fill up on greens
* Use dips such as hummus and tzatziki sparingly, because the calories can add up
* Ask if the dressing for your salad is high in fat; if you can't get plain vinegar (or a straight answer), ask for your dressing on the side and use sparingly

Ideal meal

* Order chicken souvlaki; since it is often served with rice, remember that ⅓ cup cooked rice is equal to one serving of starch
* Begin your meal with Avgolemono or a small Greek salad with dressing on the side

American Steak House

Beware of . . .

* Fatty beef cuts . . . and that includes prime rib
* Dinner rolls (they usually contain refined white flour)
* Sour cream and butter for potato fixings
* Cream-based soups such as New England clam chowder
* Anything fried (this covers an assortment of appetizers)
* Potatoes—often the size of potatoes in a restaurant are two and three times larger than a regular serving size at home

Safer to try . . .

* Lean cuts of beef
* Small butterfly filet mignon
* Skinless chicken
* Shrimp and lobster *without butter*
* Vegetable-based soups
* Shrimp cocktail

Tips . . .

* Beware of enormous portion sizes; a steak can weigh as much as 8 ounces at *minimum*
* Share a meal with someone; order one dinner and two side salads
* Ask for dressings on the side
* Split your potato with someone or take it home

Ideal meal

* Begin your meal with a small dinner salad with dressing on the side

* Use vinegar and oil
* Order a petit filet mignon (although it is a bit high in fat) with a side of vegetables
* Ask that your vegetables be prepared without sauces or butter
* Try to avoid ordering a potato or rice with your meal; if you do order a potato, split your potato with someone at your table

Seafood

Beware of. . .

* Fried fish, shrimp
* Butter sauces
* Tartar sauce
* Rice and potato dishes; these may be high in fat
* Breads
* New England clam chowder

Safer to try. . .

* Grilled fish without butter or oil
* Steamed fish
* Steamed vegetables
* Crab cocktail
* Shrimp cocktail
* Cocktail sauce—use sparingly
* Manhattan clam chowder
* Ceviche
* Bouillabaise
* Lobster without the butter (it is still wonderful)

Tips . . .

* Ordering grilled does not mean fat free . . . ask for dry fish
* Ask for all sauces on the side
* If ordering rice or potatoes, be aware of portion sizes
* Fish is always a good choice; just be careful of its preparation
* Be aware of any health risks associated with certain fish (pregnant women should avoid ordering swordfish, shark, tuna, and mackerel because of possible levels of mercury content)
* Oysters are prepared many different ways; some varieties call for butter and bread crumbs (like Rockefeller); ask that oysters be broiled with a small amount of oil and lemon

Ideal meal

* Order any type of fish you like; ask that it be prepared with a small amount of oil or dry
* Order sauces on the side
* Have extra vegetables on your plate instead of rice or potatoes
* Begin your meal with a soup (such as Manhattan clam chowder or bouillabaisse) or a salad
* A shrimp cocktail is also a good appetizer

Salad Bar

Beware of . . .

* Croutons
* Bacon bits
* Cheese (a whopping 100 calories per ounce)
* High fat, creamy dressings—2 tablespoons of Roquefort dressing can be as high as 240 calories
* Marinated artichoke hearts, olives

* Premade salads such as tuna, chicken, seafood, and egg (high in fat)
* Pasta salads made with mayonnaise

Safer to try . . .

* Lean proteins such as grilled chicken, turkey, crabmeat, fresh tuna
* Vinegar-based dressings
* Egg whites
* Kidney beans and garbanzo beans (chickpeas)
* Any and all vegetables

Tips . . .

* Load up on a variety of vegetables—add red bell peppers for color and texture, celery for crunch
* Order your dressing on the side, then dip the tines of your fork in the dressing and lightly drizzle on your salad
* Sprinkle 1 tablespoon of seeds on the salad for texture (fat calories can add up here, so moderate the amount)

Ideal meal

* Load up on any type of green vegetable
* Add tomato and onions for color
* Go easy on shredded carrots (high in sugar)
* Add egg whites and roasted chicken for a protein punch, or use tuna that is fresh and has not been mixed with mayonnaise
* Add kidney and garbanzo beans
* If you need a little crunch, try sprinkling some seeds on your salad—but go easy on this because the calories can add up quickly

* Avoid croutons
* Sprinkle your salad with vinegar and a touch of olive oil; you can use other dressings, but do so sparingly
* Use your fork to gently apply dressing to your salad

Sandwich Shops

Beware of . . .

* White refined bread
* French roll
* Croissant
* Italian deli meats such as mortadella and salami
* Cheese
* Premade salads such as tuna, chicken, seafood, and egg
* Mayonnaise

Safer to try . . .

* Whole grain bread
* Pumpernickel bread
* Sourdough bread
* Lean meats such as roasted turkey and chicken
* Mustard

Tips . . .

* Load up on vegetables; ask for extra lettuce and tomatoes
* Add pickles and peppers for zip
* Skip drizzling oil on your sandwich—try drizzling vinegar instead
* Order a side salad instead of chips (with dressing on the side)

* Ask for a side of fresh fruit
* Be aware of portion size; some submarine sandwiches are enough for two people

Ideal meal

* Roasted turkey breast on pumpernickel or sourdough bread
* Use mustard, tomato, pickles, and peppers to add flavor
* Order a side salad instead of fries, chips, coleslaw, or potato salad

Diners and Delis

Beware of . . .

* Fried foods
* High fat meats such as corned beef, pastrami, and roast beef
* Tuna salad, egg salad, chicken salad
* French fries, onion rings, potato salad, macaroni salad, coleslaw
* Large servings—meats used in sandwiches are often three and four times the amount considered a regular serving size (3 to 4 ounces)
* Refined breads
* High fat salad dressings
* Soups made with cream bases
* Big salads—chef and Cobb salads can have 1,000 calories
* High-sugar soft drinks
* Desserts

Safer to try . . .

* Lean roast turkey breast

* Grilled chicken breast sandwiches
* Fruit as a side dish or dessert
* Salads with dressing on the side
* Grilled chicken salads
* Chef salads without cheese
* Diet sodas

Tips . . .

* Order sandwiches on whole wheat, sourdough, pumpernickel, or rye breads
* Condiments on the side
* Split a sandwich or burger with a friend
* Start off with a broth-based soup to fill up
* Order sliced tomatoes instead of fries, macaroni salad, potato salad, or coleslaw
* Order a side salad first—you'll fill up faster

Ideal meal

* Order a hamburger on a whole grain bun with fixings on the side
* Order a side salad and split your hamburger with someone else or take the rest home
* Avoid cheeses and mayonnaise; this method allows you to enjoy an occasional hamburger without going overboard
* Order a grilled chicken sandwich with no cheese or mayonnaise
* Order a turkey sandwich on whole grain, pumpernickel, or sourdough bread

Breakfast and Brunch

Beware of . . .

* Eggs Benedict—hollandaise sauce is too fatty
* French toast and pancakes—too much sugar, fat, and refined carbohydrates
* Omelettes with high fat meats and cheeses
* Hash
* Potatoes
* Bacon and sausage
* Bagels and cream cheese
* Muffins
* Croissants
* Cream and sugar
* Lattes and cappuccinos
* Mixed coffee drinks

Safer to try . . .

* Egg white omelettes with extra vegetables
* Omelettes prepared with little or no oil
* Omelettes with chicken
* Whole grain cereals
* Oatmeal
* Fruit and nonfat yogurt
* Whole grain breads
* Lean ham
* Tomatoes or cottage cheese instead of potatoes
* Frittata—ask your server how it is prepared
* Lox
* Sweetener for coffee

Tips . . .

* Split an omelette with a friend and have a side of fresh fruit
* Ask your server to bring toast unbuttered
* Split a bagel with a friend—cream cheese on the side
* Ask what's in your coffee drink—these drinks often have added sugar, cream, and steamed whole milk
* If you must have pancakes, choose whole grain and top with fresh fruit; avoid syrups, which will surely spike your blood sugar levels

Ideal meal

* Egg white omelette with vegetables
* Substitute sliced tomatoes or an order of fresh fruit for potatoes
* If ordering toast or bagel, opt for pumpernickel and eat only half—or skip this all together
* Do not order fruit juice, because the carbohydrates add up quickly; go with whole fruit instead

Fast Food Restaurants

Hamburger and Chicken Joints

Beware of . . .

* Fried chicken
* Anything fried
* French fries (both high in fat and a high glycemic index factor)
* Mashed potatoes (high glycemic index factor)
* Gravy
* Biscuits
* Onion rings

* Mayonnaise
* Burgers—if you must, choose those without cheese and high fat dressings
* Nuggets (very high in fat)
* Breakfast sandwiches made with sausage and bacon (high in fat) on a croissant or a biscuit (highly refined)
* Fried fish sandwich (in some cases, this has more calories than a hamburger!)
* Milk shakes
* Regular sodas

So what's left?

Safer to try . . .

* Grilled chicken sandwich; choose whole wheat bun if available
* Chicken salads
* Side salad with dressing on the side
* Mustard
* Regular hamburger without cheese—no Super Size
* Diet sodas
* Iced tea

Tips . . .

* Some fast food places offer other items like chef salads, stuffed pitas, and tacos; watch out for hidden sources of fat in the dressings; skip ground meat tacos
* Even "healthy" chicken sandwiches can be loaded with fat; watch out for cheese, avocado, and bacon

Ideal meal

* Order a grilled chicken sandwich on a whole wheat bun

* Order without cheese and mayonnaise; use mustard instead
* Order with a side salad and a diet soft drink

Rotisserie Chicken Restaurants

Beware of...

* Dark meat
* Creamed spinach
* Macaroni and cheese
* Sautéed vegetables
* Biscuits
* White rice
* Mashed potatoes
* Soups with cream base

Safer to try...

* Light meat
* Steamed vegetables
* Baked yams, sweet potatoes
* Brown rice
* Cold vegetable salads
* Soups with broth, vegetable base

Tips...

* Ask your servers how certain dishes are prepared; for example, the vegetables at one restaurant might have butter or oil
* Remove any skin from chicken before eating; there will be inherently more fat when chicken has been cooked with the

skin on, but removing the skin before eating will save on calories and unhealthy fat

Ideal meal

* ⁕ Order chicken breast with a side of vegetables and brown rice
* ⁕ Keep in mind that one serving of rice is ⅓ cup, cooked
* ⁕ Do not eat any rolls or lavash that might come with your meal

Chapter Four

Special Situations

· · · · · · · · · · · ·

A few simple rules will help you stay within your dietary guidelines when applied to special situations such as cruises, buffets, and plane flights. When you find yourself in these potentially confining situations, it helps to either prepare ahead by bringing your own meals and snacks, or knowing how to make the best of the limited choices offered to you.

Healthy Tips in Any Situation

Some rules can be applied to virtually any situation to help you stay the course. Since they are easy to remember, and easy to apply, you'll find it to be less of an uphill struggle to maintain your diet. Such rules are particularly helpful in special situations that have already added to your stress; travel, parties, camping, and just being away from home or undergoing a change of routine under any circumstances.

Instead of expending energy trying to count each carbohydrate, you can focus a little attention on observing these simple guidelines and then get down to the task of enjoying your meal.

* Quarter Plate Rule—Restricting yourself to the point of excluding all foods is not the best approach to long-term maintenance of weight and/or healthy weight loss. It can be very hard to resist certain foods under any situation—especially holidays and vacations. The quarter plate rule is one way to allow yourself a little something without overindulging, and suffering the consequences later. First, fill your plate with an assortment of vegetables (but be aware of hidden fats used in their preparation). Then, choose a protein for one-quarter of your plate. This might include lean fish, poultry, or tofu. Finally, place a small amount of whatever else interests you on *one-quarter of your plate.* That's it. Deprivation often leads to reactionary eating, so allow yourself some flexibility without overindulging to the detriment of your health.
* No seconds please. Once you've made your plate, consider that a finished product. It is often the second and third helpings that do us in. Remember, allow some variety in your meal . . . but watch your portion sizes!
* ALWAYS be aware of the portion size. When in any dining situation, be aware that most restaurants do not give a standard portion size (that is, the size according to the USDA or ADA). There are ways to deal with this.
  —Save half your meal for another "leftover" meal (that is, why not take home half your chicken dish to use in a luncheon salad the following day?).
  —Share your meal with a friend. Order a standard dish, such as chicken, fish, or lean steak. Split each meal—halve your potato, protein, and vegetables. Then each of you should order a small dinner salad. But watch the dressing!

—Ask your server for substitutions. Get extra vegetables in place of mashed potatoes laden with butter.

—Sauces on the side, please. One tablespoon of butter is 100 calories. One tablespoon of oil is 120 calories. While some fats, such as those found in olive oil, are healthy, the calories add up quickly.

—Decline the bread basket. Some grains are considered low glycemic. Typically, the bread on the table poses two threats—most are refined and not as nutrient dense as other grains, and it is difficult to resist eating more than one serving. Add the butter and you've consumed too much of a not-so-good thing. The exception? Enjoy healthy whole grain breads and hearty fare such as pumpernickel bread.

Airborne with Diabetes

Most airlines offer diabetic meals, vegetarian meals, or "light" meals. Be forewarned about "light" meals, however; "light" doesn't always mean low calorie or—by any stretch—low in sugar or carbohydrate. When eating those little bags of nuts served on airplanes, keep in mind the "nut factor." Nuts can provide good fats, but those fats add up quickly. One ounce of nuts on average provides close to 200 calories (mostly fat), and up to 9 grams of carbohydrate.

Always call ahead to see what diabetic meals are offered. We've supplied a list of airline numbers to call to get this information. Most airlines offer diabetic meal options, as long as you call at least twenty-four hours in advance to make special arrangements.

Airline Phone Numbers

Air France	1-800-237-2747
Air New Zealand	1-800-262-1234
Air Pacific LTD	1-800-227-4446

Alaska Airlines	1-800-252-7522
American Airlines	1-800-223-5436
British Air	1-800-AIRWAYS
Continental Airlines	(310) 271-8733
Delta Airlines Inc.	1-800-221-1212
	(national/ domestic);
	1-800-241-4141 (international)

Delta offers diabetic and kosher meals. Children, toddler, and vegetarian meals are also offered as low fat.

Hawaiian Airlines	1-800-367-5320
Northwest Airlines	1-800-225-2525
Southwest Airlines	1-800-435-9792

No food is offered on longer Southwest flights, only snacks.

United Airlines	1-800-241-6522
US Airways	1-800-428-4322
Virgin Atlantic	1-800-862-8621

Cruises

Dining on cruises can be a minefield for anyone who is watching her weight and blood sugars. The variety of food choices on these "traveling cities" can be both good and bad: bad, because it's easy to consistently overindulge for however long you're sailing the seas; good, because a wealth of variety leaves room for the seafarer with diabetes to make choices. A cruise is like having your own waterborne town (only flashier!), so you should apply all of the dining out tips found in Chapters 3 and 4.

Because of the variety of options, sailing the seas shouldn't pose too many difficulties when it comes to managing your dietary needs. While temptation may run high, you do have choices; it's up to you to make prudent choices.

Most cruise lines are very accommodating in meeting the special requests of their guests. The following list of cruise lines outlines their policies in helping to meet your dietary needs. Note that the request protocols vary from one cruise line to another. Always speak to your agent to find out about specific procedures.

Cruise Lines

Carnival

Both a main seating and a late seating are available on Carnival. Requests for special dietary meals must be made by your travel agent at least two weeks prior to sailing. Carnival also suggests that you speak directly to your waiter or the headwaiter.

Celebrity Cruises

Like most cruise lines, Celebrity offers both main seating and late seating times. This is worth noting for those of you who keep a regular dining schedule. Celebrity will accommodate special dietary needs including diabetic and low cholesterol meals. Travelers must request special needs at least fifteen days prior to sailing. Contact the Special Services Department on the day of departure (or, in sailing terms, *debarking*). Contact the Restaurant Manager to confirm requests.

Crystal Cruises

This ship offers a variety of twenty-four-hour culinary experiences. Room service, per usual, is also offered. In order to have your dietary needs met, contact Crystal Cruises at least one month prior to sailing. Submit your requests in writing to the Onboard Guest Services Department. Additionally, you should contact the Food and Beverage Staff on the day you sail.

Cunard Grand Ocean Liners

Cunard Cruises, which include the *Queen Elizabeth 2* and the *Corona*, offer several culinary choices. You can choose from fine dining to casual poolside snacking. Twenty-four-hour room service is also available. Cunard requests that travelers contact the cruise line for special dietary requests at the time of booking; certainly, no later than four weeks before sailing.

Holland America

Holland America, which sails Alaska, suggests that dietary requests be made at the time of booking. This ship offers many diets for special needs. Kosher, gluten-free, and special medical diets must be pre-ordered a minimum of thirty days prior to sailing. Contact Holland America's Ship Services Department to request special meals.

Norwegian Cruise Line

Norwegian, which sails the Caribbean and Bermuda, offers open seating at breakfast, lunch, and dinner at assigned times. List your preferences at the time of booking. Ask your travel agent about requesting special dietary meals.

Orient Lines

Special dietary needs must be received in writing at least sixty days prior to sailing. Again, main and second seatings are available.

Princess Caribbean

The ocean-bound traveler will find a multitude of dining options aboard the *Princess Caribbean,* including twenty-four-hour room service. A nice feature offered by this cruise line is the individual refrigerators that can be found in each stateroom; you can save a portion of your meal for a snack later, if you choose. Contact your travel agent for more information on special dietary requests.

Princess—Mexican Riviera

Princess Cruise Line recommends that you have your travel agent specify any special dietary needs at the time of booking. A variety of dining experiences are available, including twenty-four-hour room service (in case you need a snack).

Radisson Seven Seas Cruises

Radisson Seven Seas, which sails throughout Asia, Australia, and the South Pacific, offers a variety of fine dining experiences. Onboard restaurants offer special low calorie and heart healthy selections. Twenty-four-hour room service is available, too (you never know when you'll need a snack). Special dietary requests must be made using the

Guest Information Form four weeks prior to sailing. In order to make special arrangements, contact the Reservations Department.

Renaissance Cruises

Renaissance offers several dining options. Sample menus are available through your travel agent as brochures. This line also offers a small in-room refrigerator for your convenience (in suites). Speak to your travel agent to make special arrangements with Renaissance.

Royal Caribbean International

Royal Caribbean offers a wide variety of dining experiences. As is the case with most ships, dining times vary. There is a main seating and a second seating for most meals. You should note the times in case you're taking medications; of course, Royal Caribbean also offers twenty-four-hour room service. For special needs, have your travel agent notify Royal Caribbean Reservations in writing at the time of the booking.

"All You Can Eat" Buffets, Parties, and Weddings

Because of the festive nature of celebrations, it is easy to lead yourself down the path of self-indulgence—but resist! Keep in mind these simple guidelines, which will allow you to enjoy yourself by partaking of the culinary aspects of the festivities while preventing you from going to extremes. The cardinal rule of everything in moderation especially applies here; by allowing yourself enough leeway in your diet to not feel deprived and still staying within a safe dietary zone, you'll have an easier time staying the course and avoid binge eating.

* Always fill one-half of your plate with a green salad. Fill one-quarter of the plate with protein, such as chicken or fish. Fill the last one-quarter of the plate with vegetables and/or a grain. Remember, this is the *quarter plate rule.*

* Avoid breads, muffins, cakes, and cookies. If you must have a little cake, consume a small amount and be sure that you have had a balanced meal beforehand.
* Eat crudités, but go easy on any dipping sauces. Vegetables are a great way to fill up before, during, and after a meal.
* Be careful of dishes that are prepared in sauces. Starch or sugar may be added to sauces as well as a lot of fat. Avoid dishes like enchiladas or casseroles. These can be laden with hidden calories.
* Take advantage of seafood buffets. Shrimp and crab make wonderful appetizers without consuming a lot of calories. Squeeze fresh lemon juice on the seafood and go easy on the cocktail sauce.
* Choose lean protein dishes like chicken or fish. Choose proteins that are prepared without sauces such as grilled or roasted chicken, beef, and fish.
* Beware of the diabetic desserts that many buffets offer! These can still be high in carbohydrates. Sugar-free may mean that the dessert is sucrose free, but not necessarily free of other forms of sugar such as fructose.
* Select fresh fruit as a dessert.
* Be conscious of the dietary effects of champagne and other alcoholic beverages. Remember that alcohol will affect your blood sugar levels and that its consumption is not recommended. If you choose to consume alcohol, one drink should be counted as two fat exchanges.

Conventioneering and Being Hotel Bound with Diabetes

The most sage advice we can offer is this: Call ahead to your hotel and ask what services are available. Generally, for a convention, there is a set menu. Typically, there is a vegetarian meal and/or a diabetic meal. However, this doesn't mean that the food offered will fit your specific needs. The following steps will ensure that you get your dietary needs met.

* Call the hotel and/or organization holding the convention. Ask for a detailed menu and, most importantly, a list of scheduled times for dining. Meal times are particularly important for the person with diabetes who is on medications.
* Ask for any meals that fit your needs. Be sure to have a confirmation number to guarantee that you receive an appropriate meal per your specifications. Often, during the hustle and bustle, orders can be lost. Double-check first thing in the morning before your day begins to ensure the hotel or organization remembers to make special preparations.
* Have portable snacks that you can take with you. During breaks, snacks are often provided, but these are generally high sugar foods such as cookies and crackers. Bring the following items with you in case of an emergency:

Low-carbohydrate protein bars
Part-skim mozzarella string cheese
Apples
A single serving of nuts

* If room service is available, order breakfast first. Typical breakfast items include Continental-type items such as muffins, sweet rolls, and croissants. Many hotels have a coffee shop that is accessible. Order a breakfast rich in complex carbohydrates and protein to keep your blood sugars even and sustained.

● ● ●

In the Wild

We all have fond memories of sitting around the campfire making s'mores, swapping scary stories, making more s'mores, pitching our tents, making more s'mores . . .

You get the picture. With our high-tech world, we can transport a gourmet kitchen with us when we camp; these days, getting the right food is not so difficult. As in any situation, when it comes to camping, preparation is *always* the key.

* Bring a lot of snack items. Individual serving size packages of nuts are great for the energy needed to hike and play. Individual packages of string cheese and protein bars (many of these are made with sugar alcohol, which may or may not affect an individual's blood sugar) are also handy snack items. Turkey or salmon jerky offer a change of pace, as well.
* If grilling, bring along whole grain buns for hot dogs and hamburgers. Choose chicken or turkey franks, which are generally lower in fat. If storage of meats is a concern, precook meats before storing in refrigerated containers. This works well for chicken breasts.
* Bring whole pieces of fruit. These are easy to throw in a backpack if you go for a hike.
* Bring individual servings of oatmeal for your morning meals. Don't load up on the high-in-sugar varieties, however. You can package natural, "old-fashioned" oat cereal yourself in plastic bags, and flavor it with natural fruit.
* Chips and similar junk foods can sabotage your efforts to maintain blood sugar levels and overall weight. Try cut-up veggies dipped in light dip.
* Bring a lot of water and keep drinking. Dehydration is always a concern, especially in high altitudes.

Chapter Five

Everyday Menus and Holidays

Everyday Menus

A word about the following menus—for most we used the principles of low glycemic eating. You should note that while, in most cases, the numbers indicate that there will not be a rapid glycemic response, individuals can have different responses to the same food item. For example, while one individual may not have an elevated blood sugar from eating nonfat yogurt (a food with a low glycemic value), another might experience a rise in blood sugar levels. Please be aware of how your individual body responds to certain foods. In this way, you can take charge of your health.

Each day's menu provides approximately 1,400 to 1,550 calories with an *average* of 130 grams of carbohydrate. Because we are also sensitive to the amount of carbohydrate, limited portions of starch have been added with some listed as *optional*. These menus are reduced both in calories and carbohydrates and are beneficial for those who are trying to achieve some weight loss.

* There are at least two servings of fruit each day to meet the recommendations of the Food Guide Pyramid.
* Starches are limited, but for those included, consideration was given to glycemic index values.
* Some dairy items are included daily, including milk, yogurt, and cheese. If you are sensitive to dairy products, omit these options.
* Choose nuts or lean turkey (as an example) as a snack option in limited quantities. Nuts, per ounce, provide an average of 170 calories. Be careful of amounts consumed.
* If calories are a consideration and more are needed, we suggest increasing vegetables and lean proteins such as fish and chicken.
* Calories add up in salad dressings. We suggest using a vinegar with a bit of olive oil instead of store-bought dressings, which are often high in fat and calories. Green salads provide bulk and nutrients that are needed without impacting blood sugar levels. The addition of oils for either cooking or salads will add to the amount of calories consumed.
* All menu items in italics will be found in chapter 6, "Recipes."

Day 1

Breakfast:
3 egg-white omelette with ½ cup green pepper and mushrooms
1 cup raspberries

Snack:
1 ounce nuts

Lunch:

1 cup vegetable soup

Turkey sandwich on 100% whole-grain wheat bread (Oroweat Light)

Snack:

½ cup cut vegetables, raw

1 ounce cheese

Dinner:

Green salad

Chicken Florentine

1 cup vegetables, such as steamed cauliflower

Dessert/Snack:

1 small pear, cored, cut, with a dash of cinnamon

½ cup nonfat yogurt, plain

Day 2

Breakfast:

½ cup steel-cut oats, cooked

1 slice sourdough toast

1 tablespoon peanut butter

Snack:

1 small apple

½ cup cottage cheese

Lunch:

Gorgonzola, Walnut, Pear, and Grilled Chicken Salad

Whole grain roll, small

Snack:

1 mozzarella string cheese stick

1 cup low-sodium broth

½ cup cut vegetables, raw

Dinner:

Shrimp Etouffee

½ cup brown rice (optional)

1 cup broccoli, steamed

Green salad

Dessert/Snack:

Sugar-free Popsicle

15 cherries

Day 3

Breakfast:

⅓ cup bran cereal (All-Bran or Bran Buds)

½ cup skim milk

½ cup strawberries, sliced

Snack:

½ cup nonfat, fruit flavored yogurt or plain, with articial
  sweetener

1 peach

Lunch:

Greek Salad for One

Snack:

½ whole wheat pita

1 ounce spreadable light cheese (Laughing Cow)

Dinner:

Stuffed Green Pepper

½ cup brown rice (optional)

Green salad

Dessert/Snack:

½ cup nonfat cottage cheese

½ medium peach

Day 4

Breakfast:

3 egg-white omelette with ½ ounce feta cheese, ½ cup mushrooms,
and spinach

½ cup mixed fruit

Snack:

1 slice pumpernickel toast

1 tablespoon cream cheese, low fat

1 thin slice tomato

Lunch:

2 cups *Lentil Soup*

Green Fiesta Salad

Snack:

1 cup soy milk or nonfat milk

1 cup strawberries

(blend for fruit smoothie)

Dinner:

Grilled Portobello Mushroom and Asparagus Salad

Basic Marinated Chicken on the Grill

Dessert/Snack:

Sugar-free Jell-O

1 tablespoon nonfat whipped topping (Cool Whip)

Day 5

Breakfast:

2 slices 100% whole-grain wheat bread (Oroweat Light)

½ cup nonfat cottage cheese

dash cinnamon and sweetener

(broil to create mock pastry)

Snack:

1 ounce nuts

1 plum

Lunch:

Turkey Chili

Green Fiesta Salad

1 small apple

Snack:

1 cup cut vegetables, raw

1 ounce cheese

Dinner:

Avocado and Spinach Salad

Broiled salmon (or other favorite fish)

½ cup rice, converted or parboiled

Dessert/Snack:

Sugar-free Popsicle

Day 6

Breakfast:

1 cup steel-cut oats, cooked

½ cup soy milk or ½ cup nonfat milk

½ cup berries

Snack:

½ medium apple

1 tablespoon peanut butter

Lunch:

½ cup cooked pasta (linguini, fettuccini)

1 5-ounce chicken breast, grilled

1½ cups cooked vegetables (sprinkle with Parmesan cheese and
1 tablespoon olive oil)

Snack:

½ medium grapefruit

Dinner:

Shark Fillet in Wine and Dill Sauce

1 cup steamed green beans

Large green salad

Dessert/Snack:

Sugar-free Jell-O

1 tablespoon nonfat whipped topping (Cool Whip)

Day 7

Breakfast:

1 cup soy milk or 1 cup nonfat milk

1 scoop protein powder of choice (low carbohydrate variety)

½ medium peach

½ cup raspberries

(blend for smoothie)

1 slice pumpernickel bread, toasted

Snack:

1 ounce nuts

Lunch:

Stir-Fried Beef Salad

Whole grain roll, small

Snack:

1 mozzarella string cheese stick

1 cup cut vegetables, raw

Dinner:

Steamed Fish in Lime Essence

½ cup brown rice

Ratatouille

Dessert/Snack:

15 cherries

Holidays

Without question, the holidays present many challenges when it comes to watching your blood sugar and/or weight. There is always a wide assortment of goodies and foods that are rich in both fat and sugar. In the celebratory atmosphere of seasonal holidays, you may find yourself thinking, what does it matter if you break the rules just once?

To make a point, a typical Thanksgiving dinner with all the fixings (turkey, potatoes, candied yams, stuffing, peas and carrots, rolls, cranberries, and one piece of pie) can be as high as 1,500 to 2,000 calories. This, of course, is if you don't pay attention to both preparation and portion sizes of food.

However, don't fear—it is possible to enjoy the typical fare during the holidays, with a few preparatory changes and substitutions. We've provided menus for the following holidays:

Valentine's Day for Two
Passover

Easter

Fourth of July

Thanksgiving

Hanukkah

Christmas

New Year's Eve

One of the biggest temptations during the holidays is to adopt the mind-set of "Oh, Christmas only comes once a year, so I can indulge." You should toss this logic out the window for a couple of reasons. First, holidays will always come back. You don't have to gorge on these foods because you might not ever see them again—you will. Second, you *can* enjoy the holidays without overindulging.

There may be an instant gratification factor, but once the calories have been consumed, there is no turning back. Your sugars may run high, you'll pack on the pounds, and in all likelihood, your temporary enjoyment of the foods will be more than offset by your guilt and the negative consequences for your overall health.

Distract yourself from eating by engaging in other activities. Try going for a walk with family or friends after a large meal. Engage in conversation, tell stories, laugh, and play. Holidays shouldn't be about tasting all the new desserts that year.

Okay—we know what you're probably saying: "But eating Aunt So-and-So's pecan pie is a tradition." Perhaps, to complicate matters, you are not even in charge of the menu. Someone else is cooking for you and adding all the fat and sugar they want. Fair enough. There are many visual and olfactory triggers during the holidays . . . you *see* your favorite cookies on the table and you *smell* your favorite stuffing as it passes you by. You might give anything for some kugel. There are ways to modify your mentality and old habits; it's worth making the effort—your body will thank you for it.

Often, food is part of the ritual, as it is during Passover dinner. We aren't suggesting that you not partake in a ritual; just be aware of the quantity of food you consume and how it is prepared. Here are some suggestions to help you through each holiday:

* Be aware of portion sizes.
* If temptation is too high, allow yourself a small amount. Deprivation often leads to reactionary eating; that is, you were fine during dinner, but now that the dishes are cleaned and the food is in the refrigerator, *you have to have it . . . now!* This is all too common, and often leads to feelings of guilt and shame. Don't put yourself in a position where you are tempted to overcompensate for abstaining from eating your favorite foods. If you want something, then have it . . . only, have a little.
* *Follow the quarter plate rule.* One-quarter of your plate can be reserved for all the "questionable" items, such as candied yams, mashed potatoes (remember that these have a high glycemic index), and stuffing. One-quarter of your plate is for protein (that is, turkey, brisket, or ham). The remaining half should be full of vegetables (ideally, without butter) or salad.
* Offer to bring an item such as crudités or deviled eggs with light mayo. Or bring a lovely garden salad, served with a light vinaigrette. If there is a food item available that is both good for you and that you enjoy, it will be easier for you to fill up on that and be less inclined to indulge in unhealthy alternatives.
* Fill up on nonalcoholic drinks such as club soda with a twist of lime, orange, or lemon. Enjoy sugar-free hot apple cider. Add a cinnamon stick, and you have a great drink.
* When drinking alcoholic beverages, remember that booze adds up . . . fast. Alcohol can actually lower blood sugar in some individuals. Treat one drink as two exchanges of fat (now it doesn't sound so good, right?). Remember that drinking adds unwanted calories and lowers your resolve to limit your consumption of both alcohol and food. Drink responsibly.

* If wine is part of a holiday ritual, as it is during Passover, consume as little as possible, due to its high level of carbohydrate.

In the following section, we provide several holiday menus. Recipes for each menu can be found in the recipe section of the book. As a rule of thumb, we present each menu with a few considerations:

* Each food item was selected with consideration for its glycemic index value.
* We provide recommended serving sizes; however, a specific breakdown of calories is not included. By utilizing the exchange lists or by referencing the food composition tables, you can determine the amount of carbohydrates and fat you're consuming.
* The recipes included here are modified versions of old favorites; they are written and revised with consideration for fat and sugar values. We want you to be able to enjoy holiday meals that are as close as possible to your traditional favorites; fortunately, you can eat, be merry, and still adhere to a diabetes-conscientious diet.

Valentine's Day for Two

Valentine's Day leads to a night of romance, and is characterized by the decadent flavors of rich foods and sinful desserts. This simple menu offers full-bodied flavors without the high calories from either fat or sugar. Gorgonzola, while not a low fat cheese, offers a powerful flavor to a typical dinner salad. Cordon bleu, which is traditionally very rich with its blend of ham and cheese, is offered here in a lighter variety. Roasted Portobello mushrooms provide a heartiness to the meal. Finally, strawberries are a sweet alternative to typical chocolate fare.

Appetizer

Gorgonzola and Walnut Side Salad
(with light vinaigrette)

Entrée

Chicken Cordon Bleu (Mock)
Roasted Portobello Mushrooms

Dessert

Fresh strawberries and cream

Easter

Easter is a wonderful time to get together with friends and family. We've included recipes for a traditional Easter dinner that will still meet all your diabetic needs.

Appetizer

Deviled Eggs Light

Entrée

Ham
Green Beans, Steamed

Dessert

Angel Food Cake with Fresh Fruit

Passover

Our friends Rami Aisic and Mason Sommers were kind enough to prepare the following menu for a traditional Passover Seder. This holiday celebrates the victory of the Jews over the Pharaoh as they were freed from slavery in Egypt. The meal, which involves partaking in certain foods from the Seder plate, retells the story of the exodus. Following this portion of the Passover meal, foods such as brisket or roast chicken is served. We included this portion of the meal because of its symbolic significance.

* Maror (bitter herbs). Horseradish is often used for this, symbolizing the bitterness of the Egyptian slavery.
* Z'roah (shankbone). This is symbolic of the paschal lamb offered as the Passover sacrifice in biblical times. Vegetarian households often use beets for the shankbone, the red being a symbol of the blood of the lamb, used to mark the doorposts of the Jewish houses in order for the Angel of Death to "pass over" those homes and afflict only the Egyptians.
* Charoset (apples, nuts, and spices). These are ground together, often with wine, symbolic of the mortar used by the Hebrew slaves to build Egyptian structures. This is sweet, as a symbol that even during the time there was hardship for the Jewish slaves, God's kindness made their lives somewhat bearable.
* Karpas (green vegetable). Usually parsley, it is dipped into salt water during the Seder. The green vegetable is symbolic of continued life, harvest, and rebirth of a new season, and the salt water represents the tears shed during slavery.
* Beitzah (roasted egg). This is symbolic of sacrifice, as well as a traditional symbol of mourning.

* Chazeret (bitter vegetable or horseradish). This is not used in all communities. Some have five elements on the Seder plate, and some include this as a sixth. This is used because the Seder calls for bitter herbs (plural), so a second bitter vegetable meets that requirement.
* Matzoh (unleavened bread). This is another main symbol of Passover, made from flour and water that has not had time to ferment, or rise. Matzoh is symbolic of the rush in which the Jews left Egypt prior to the exodus, and did not have time to let the dough rise in the making of the bread they took with them.

Fourth of July

Ahh . . . the good old-fashioned barbeque, and all its accoutrements—
creamy salads, chips and dips, desserts all around. Here we offer an
alternative to high calorie cuisine. Enjoy a healthy meal that has been
prepared on the grill. Load up on salad and enjoy a fresh fruit kabob
made with seasonal fruits. Finally, in the spirit of '76, a red, white, and
blue parfait for dessert. Feeling overwhelmed by the variety of foods
around? Remember the quarter plate rule. Drink plenty of water or
sugar free beverages. Get involved in activities to stay away from the
tempting foods. Set off fireworks and celebrate your ability to take
care of yourself and your health!

Entrée

Marinated Chicken on the Grill
Grilled Corn
Green Fiesta Salad
Fruit Kabobs

Dessert

Red, White, and Blue Parfaits

Thanksgiving

This is one holiday that can certainly impact blood sugar levels, if you aren't cautious. Images of standing in the kitchen surrounded by friends and family while the meal is being prepared come to mind. How easy it is to pick at all sorts of tantalizing treats. Then comes the main meal. Pass the mashed potatoes and gravy—and extra stuffing. Here are some relatively good alternatives to the typical fare shared at Thanksgiving dinner. Remember that the calories can still add up significantly, so watch portion sizes. Half of one cup is a serving size for both stuffing and mashed sweet potatoes. The same holds true for roasted new potatoes. You might think about sampling a bit of each rather than consuming a great deal of starch. Load up on the vegetables and eat plenty of white meat turkey (without gravy). Above all, pay more attention to the wonderful company of family and friends than on all the food that abounds.

Appetizer

Crudités with low-calorie, low-fat dressing

Entrée

Herbed Turkey
Oven-Roasted New Potatoes
Mashed Sweet Potatoes
Steamed Broccoli Florets
Whole grain rolls

Dessert

Mock Pumpkin Chiffon Pie

Hanukkah

The name *Hanukkah* comes from the rededication of the Holy Temple in Jerusalem after its destruction. During the war at that time, no oil was available for light, heat, or cooking. One small container of oil was found which had enough oil to last only one day, but it miraculously lasted for eight days, by which time the war was won. The Jews were able to clean up the Temple and rededicate it as a place of prayer.

So what types of foods are consumed? There are no standardized meals to make note of, but there are a couple of foods that are consumed because of the symbolic meaning. Jelly doughnuts and latkes (potato pancakes) often accompany meals served during the eight days of Hanukkah. Both require the use of oil in preparation, as a symbol for the oil needed historically.

Clearly, eating jelly doughnuts and latkes will not aid in maintaining healthy blood sugar levels. If you must partake of these traditional foods, do so sparingly and only when a meal is available that is balanced with protein. One 3-ounce latke contains 20 grams of carbohydrate and 190 calories. The fat content is very high. There are variations on the traditional potato latke, but all of them have high glycemic values because of their preparation.

Christmas

Once again, a holiday such as this presents many challenges when it comes to maintaining a healthy, balanced dietary intake. Homemade cookies, candies, and other assorted treats are spread out on tabletops while meals are being prepared. Expensive chocolates are passed from home to home as a gesture of kindness—and lead to tremendous temptations. Once more, remember to load up on vegetables and allow a small space on your plate for other foods. If you feel like you have to have a "little something" to snack on, keep yourself occupied. Play with someone's new toy, keep busy, and enjoy your holiday.

Appetizer

Spicy Tomato soup

Entrée

Beef Tenderloin with Pepper
Lightly Sautéed Spinach with Garlic
Brown Rice with Herbs and Mushrooms

Dessert

Chocolate Cheesecake

New Year's Eve Celebration

New Year's Eve is a time for celebration and resolutions. You do not want to break your resolve to eat healthily by overindulging in party fare that is high in calories and low in nutritional value. This is a special evening and calls for a special meal. Perfect for either a small gathering of friends or for an intimate dinner for two, take in the New Year with a delightful meal that takes care of all the senses.

Appetizer

Shrimp cocktail

Entrée

Salmon with Basil Pesto Marinade
Fettuccine and Spinach
Field greens with balsamic vinegar dressing

Dessert

Vanilla Ice Milk with Baked Pears

Chapter Six

Recipes

● ● ● ● ● ● ● ● ● ● ● ● ●

Following are some of our favorite recipes, culled from our own kitchens and those of our friends and families, and from some of the best diabetic cookbooks.

When it comes to cooking, we don't always measure herbs and spices to the teaspoon—so feel free to add these for added flavor until you get the desired taste. Don't, however, use this method of measurement when it comes to dietary fats. Use oils sparingly and use nonstick cooking spray as an alternative to oil for recipes that call for sautéing.

Soups and Salads

Spicy Tomato Soup

serves 8

¾ cup onion, finely chopped
2 stalks celery, chopped
I tablespoon olive oil
2 quarts tomato juice
2 teaspoons low sodium beef-flavored bouillon
granules
2 teaspoons Worcestershire sauce
2 teaspoons Dijon mustard
¼ teaspoon hot sauce
Lemon slices (optional)
Basil, fresh

Sauté onion and celery in oil until transparent. Add tomato juice and next four ingredients. Bring to a boil; reduce heat, and simmer for 10 minutes. Garnish with lemon slices and fresh basil.

Chicken Soup

4–5   pounds chicken pieces (thighs, back, wings)

10   cups water

6   whole peppercorns

2–3   onions, cut into eighths

6–7   carrots, cut into big pieces

6   celery sticks, cut into pieces

5   sprigs fresh parsley

2   bay leaves

1   sprig fresh thyme

1   whole clove

1   clove garlic

2   sprigs fresh dill

        Salt and pepper

Place chicken in pot, add water and remaining ingredients. Bring to a boil. Cover, lower heat to simmer and leave for at least 2 hours. Skim top to remove fat and residue. Once cooked (you can simmer it on the stove up to 3 hours), strain through cheesecloth or fine strainer. To remove excess fat, refrigerate overnight; when fat rises, it will harden and then can be easily removed.

Spinach Borscht

serves 4

I   package frozen chopped spinach
4   cups water
I   large onion, cut fine
I   level teaspoon salt, or to taste
I   small lemon, juiced
    Sour cream
    Cucumber, chopped
    Pepper
    Green onions, chopped

Bring first 5 ingredients to a boil, then reduce heat to simmer for 15 to 20 minutes, or until onions and spinach are cooked. For serving, blend with sour cream, chopped cucumber, and pepper to taste. Garnish with chopped green onions.

Vegetable Soup*

serves approximately 5

4   cups homemade chicken, beef, vegetable, or
    turkey stock
I   16-ounce can tomatoes
½   cup onions, chopped
½   cup carrots, thinly sliced
½   cup celery, diagonally sliced
½   cup green pepper, coursely chopped
½   teaspoon salt
2   tablespoons fresh lemon juice
5   whole peppercorns
½   teaspoon basil leaves, dried
¼   teaspoon hot pepper sauce
½   cup small pasta, uncooked

Combine all ingredients except pasta in a 3- to 4-quart pot. Bring to a boil, cover, and simmer gently for 1 hour. Stir occasionally to break up tomatoes into bite-sized pieces. Add pasta and cook for 5 to 7 minutes, until done. (Serving size is 1½ cups)

Reproduced with permission from Gloria Loring.

Lentil Soup*

4   cups chicken stock

2   cups water

¼   cup red wine

1   cup dry lentils

½   cup long-grain brown rice

1   16-ounce can tomatoes, chopped

1   bay leaf

¼   cup fresh parsley, chopped

1   teaspoon ground cumin

1   carrot, sliced

1   onion, chopped

1   celery stalk, sliced

2   garlic cloves, minced or pressed

½   lemon, juiced

1   bunch (6–8 ounces) fresh spinach, cleaned and steamed

Combine all ingredients except spinach in a 3- to 4-quart saucepan and bring to a boil. Reduce heat and cover. Simmer for 20 to 25 minutes or until lentils and rice are tender. Cut spinach across the leaves in long, thin shreds. Add to soup and simmer for 5 minutes. Remove bay leaf and serve. (Serving size is 1 cup.)

Reproduced with permission from Gloria Loring.

Greek Lemon Soup

serves 6 to 8

7   cups chicken broth

½   teaspoon ground pepper

¼   cup orzo or rice
     (Option: Omit rice or orzo altogether, or use
     brown rice.)

3   eggs

¼   cup fresh lemon juice

2   cups cooked chicken, chopped

I   tablespoon fresh dill, chopped

2   tablespoons fresh chives, chopped

½   lemon, sliced thin for garnish

In a 3- to 4-quart pan, bring broth and pepper to a boil. Add orzo or rice and cook accordingly (less time for orzo, about 18 to 20 minutes for rice). If not using orzo or rice, skip this step. In a small bowl, whisk eggs with lemon juice. Blend well. Add I cup hot broth. Over low heat, add egg mixture to large pan of broth. Stir constantly for 2 minutes. Add chicken, dill, and chives. Serve and garnish with lemon slices.

Gorgonzola and Walnut Side Salad

serves **4**

1	large bunch mixed field greens (if purchasing prepackaged, use two bags)
¼	cup low calorie raspberry-balsamic vinaigrette (try Rising Sun Farms)
2	large Roma tomatoes, chopped
½	cup walnuts, chopped
4	tablespoons Gorgonzola cheese, crumbled

In large bowl, toss vinaigrette with field greens. Arrange tomatoes, and sprinkle walnuts and cheese on salad.

Green Fiesta Salad

serves 10 to 12

This is a perfect salad for a large group; it makes a nice presentation, in addition to its healthy attributes.

3	heads romaine lettuce, washed and torn
1	large cucumber, sliced
4	large Roma tomatoes, sliced
2	large carrots, peeled and julienned
1	small red onion, thinly sliced
1	medium red bell pepper, slivered
1	medium green bell pepper, slivered
½	cup garbanzo beans, rinsed
½	cup kidney beans, rinsed

Toss ingredients in bowl. Serve with Zangy Tangy Vinaigrette.

Zangy Tangy Vinaigrette

serves 10 to 12

½	cup olive oil (approximately 8 teaspoons)
1	cup white balsamic vinegar
3	tablespoons spicy Dijon mustard
½	tablespoon fresh basil
½	tablespoon dried oregano
1	teaspoon garlic salt
1	teaspoon fresh ground pepper

Mix together all ingredients; serving size is 2 tablespoons.

Greek Salad for One

serves 1

3–4 cups lettuce

¼ cup red onion, chopped

3 Kalamata olives, pitted and chopped

1 large Roma tomato, sliced

¼ medium cucumber, sliced

1 tablespoon olive oil

2 tablespoons wine vinegar

4 ounces chicken breast, cubed

1 tablespoon feta cheese

Salt and pepper

In medium bowl, combine lettuce, onion, olives, tomato, and cucumber. Toss with oil and vinegar. Add chicken and feta cheese. Add salt and pepper if desired.

Stir-Fried Beef Salad

serves 4

¼   cup low-sodium soy sauce

2   tablespoons sherry

1   packet NutraSweet, or other sweetener

1   large garlic clove, minced

¼   teaspoon ground ginger

12   ounces lean beef (sirloin, flank) cut into
      thin strips
      Nonstick cooking spray

2   cups mushrooms, sliced

1   small bunch green onions, diced

1   red bell pepper, sliced

¾   pound Boston or Bibb lettuce, washed,
      dried, torn

Mix soy sauce, sherry, sweetener, garlic, and ginger in large bowl. Add beef. Marinate for at least 30 minutes, or overnight. Heat large skillet or wok. Spray with nonstick cooking spray. Add mushrooms, onions, and peppers. Cook until tender. Remove from heat. Add beef. Cook until brown or desired doneness, approximately 3 minutes. Mix beef with vegetables. Serve over bed of lettuce.

Tex-Mex Salad

4	boneless, skinless chicken breasts
	Nonstick cooking spray
¼	cup lime juice
1	teaspoon chili powder
1	teaspoon cumin
	Salt and pepper
2	cups black beans, rinsed and drained
2	cups corn, rinsed and drained
1	cup spicy salsa
¾	pound Boston or Bibb lettuce
1	avocado, pitted and cubed
½	cup cheddar cheese

Chicken can be prepared on the grill or over the stove. Spray skillet with nonstick cooking spray. Add chicken to skillet. Add lime juice, chili powder, cumin, and pepper (add more for more punch!). Salt to taste. Cook for 5 minutes. Turn chicken and cook for another 5 minutes (approximately) or until chicken is done. Remove from heat. In large bowl, mix beans, corn, and salsa. Toss. Cut chicken into small chunks. Add to mixture. Serve over lettuce. Add avocado and cheese to salad.

Mushroom and Pignoli (Pine Nut) Salad

serves **4**

1	tablespoon olive oil
1	red onion, diced
15	mushrooms, sliced
1	clove garlic, minced
	Pepper
4	tablespoons pine nuts
2	bunches spinach, rinsed, drained, torn
1½	tablespoons raspberry vinegar

In large skillet, add oil. Sautée onion, mushrooms, garlic, and pepper until mushrooms are brown and onions are tender. Remove from heat. Add pine nuts and toss. Toss with spinach and vinegar.

Warm Goat Cheese (Chèvre) Salad

serves 2

1	tablespoon lemon juice
1	tablespoon white balsamic vinegar
1	tablespoon olive oil
⅓	pound field greens
2	ounces goat cheese
4	tablespoons walnuts, finely chopped
1	tablespoon walnut oil

Mix lemon juice, white balsamic vinegar, and oil in small bowl. Toss greens with dressing. Cut goat cheese into thin slices. Coat cheese with chopped walnuts. Add walnut oil to large skillet. Place cheese in skillet and warm until cheese begins to melt. Remove from heat and place on greens.

Avocado and Spinach Salad

¼   cup red wine vinegar
¼   teaspoon dried tarragon
¼   teaspoon grainy mustard
¼   cup olive oil
¾   pound spinach, washed, rinsed, torn
1½ avocados, peeled, pitted, cubed
¼   cup black olives, chopped
¼   cup red onion, diced
¼   cup mandarin orange slices

Mix vinegar, tarragon, mustard, and oil in small bowl. Set aside. In large bowl, toss together remaining ingredients. Add dressing and toss before serving.

Gorgonzola, Walnut, Pear, and Grilled Chicken Salad

serves 4

4   grilled chicken breasts
¼   cup raspberry vinegar
2   tablespoons olive oil
     Pepper
¾   pound romaine lettuce, washed, dried, torn
2   ounces Gorgonzola cheese, crumbled
I   ounce walnuts, chopped
I   large pear, cut into 8 slices

Prepare Basic Marinated Chicken on the Grill, page II9. (This can be done ahead of time and breasts can be chilled.) Slice breasts into I-inch-thick pieces. Set aside. Whisk vinegar, oil, and pepper together in small bowl. Toss together lettuce, cheese, and walnuts. Serve with sliced chicken breast on top. Garnish with sliced pear.

Smoked Gouda, Apple, and Pecan Salad

serves 4

4	grilled chicken breasts
¼	cup white balsamic vinegar
2	tablespoons olive oil
¼	teaspoon dried basil
¼	teaspoon dried oregano
¼	teaspoon dried sage
	Pepper
¾	pound field greens
2	ounces smoked Gouda cheese, cubed
I	ounce pecans, chopped
I	medium apple, diced (Granny Smith provides a nice tart flavor that balances the sweet flavor of the pecans)

Prepare Basic Marinated Chicken on the Grill, page 119. (This can be done ahead of time and breasts can be chilled.) Slice breasts into 1-inch-thick pieces. Set aside. Whisk vinegar, oil, basil, oregano, sage, and pepper in a small bowl. Set aside. In large bowl, mix together greens, cheese, pecans, and apple. Toss with dressing. Serve with sliced chicken breast on top.

Grilled Portobello Mushroom and Asparagus Salad*

serves 6

2   ounces (3 cups) leaf lettuce
2   ounces (3 cups) mesclun-type mix of young greens
I   medium-size shallot
I   teaspoon Dijon mustard
3   tablespoons sherry wine vinegar
I   tablespoon lemon juice
I   teaspoon fresh thyme leaves
4   tablespoons extra-virgin olive oil
    Pinch of salt and freshly ground black pepper
I   pound Portobello mushrooms, stems removed
I   pound thick asparagus, woody ends removed
    Vegetable oil to brush on grill

Preheat a gas grill to medium-high or build a fire in a kettle grill. Wash, dry, and tear up lettuces. Place in large salad bowl and set aside. Place the shallot, mustard, vinegar, lemon juice, and thyme in blender. Add 3 tablespoons oil as you are blending. Season with salt and pepper. Brush mushrooms and asparagus with remaining olive oil and sprinkle with salt and pepper. Brush the grill lightly with vegetable oil. Put mushrooms on the grill, turning occasionally. Add asparagus spears, rolling frequently. Grill mushrooms for about 10 to 14 minutes. Grill asparagus for about 6 to 8 minutes. Drizzle dressing over greens and toss. Cut mushrooms and asparagus into I-inch lengths. Add to salad.

Printed with permission by McGraw-Hill. Patti A. Bess, Vegetarian Barbeque & Other Pleasures of the Harvest, *1999, pp. 212–213.*

Seafood Entrées

Shark Fillets in Wine
and Dill Sauce

serves 2

2	tablespoons olive oil
2	shark fillets, 6–7 ounces each
	Salt and pepper
½	lemon, juiced
3	tablespoons fresh dill, crushed
⅓	cup dry white wine

Add oil to large skillet. Heat over medium heat. Salt and pepper shark to taste. Add to skillet. Squeeze juice of lemon over fish. Sprinkle with dill and add wine. Cook for 3 to 4 minutes. Turn and cook for 3 to 4 minutes or until fish flakes easily with a fork.

Seafood Stew*

I   cup chopped onion

I   clove garlic, minced

2   cups fresh tomatoes, chopped

2   10½-ounce cans condensed beef broth (preferably low sodium)

½   cup cream sherry

4   lemon slices

3   whole allspice

I   bay leaf

I   pound skinned fish fillets

I   pound shrimp, deveined

I   dozen clams or I 10-ounce can chopped clams,
undrained

¼   cup Parmesan cheese, grated

Simmer onion, garlic, tomatoes, beef broth, sherry, lemon slices, and seasonings, uncovered, for 30 minutes. Cut fish fillets into large chunks. Add fish, shrimp, and clams to pot. Simmer 15 to 20 minutes or until clams open. Top with grated Parmesan cheese. Serve with salad and garlic bread. (Serving size is 1½ cups.)

Reproduced with permission from Gloria Loring.

Steamed Fish in Lime Essence

serves **4**

In order to prepare this meal, you must have the proper equipment. A steamer rack and a sizable pan to fit the steamer rack is necessary.

4	tilapia fillets (any fish can be used), 5–6 ounces each
1	lime
¼	cup shallots
½	cup fresh cilantro, chopped
	Pepper

Arrange fish on the rack over boiling water. Squeeze juice of lime over fish. Cover fish with chopped shallots and chopped cilantro. Pepper to taste. Cover and steam for approximately 7 minutes, or until fish flakes with a fork and appears opaque.

Shrimp Étouffée

serves 4 to 6

Nonstick cooking spray

2   cloves minced garlic

4   green onions, chopped

¼   cup chicken stock (or vegetable stock)

1   bay leaf

½   lemon, juiced

Salt and pepper to taste

1   teaspoon rosemary

¼   cup white wine

2   pounds raw shrimp, peeled and deveined

¼   cup chopped parsley

1½   cups brown rice, cooked

Coat medium skillet with nonstick cooking spray. Add garlic and green onions; sauté until soft. Add stock, bay leaf, lemon juice, salt and pepper, rosemary, and ½ of the wine. Simmer for 10 minutes. Remove bay leaf, add shrimp, and continue cooking for 20 minutes. Add remaining wine and parsley. Serve over rice.

Broiled, Marinated Halibut

serves 4

Nonstick cooking spray

6 ounces fresh mushrooms, sliced

2 teaspoons Dijon style mustard

2 tablespoons lemon juice

¼ cup white cooking wine

4 halibut steaks (about ⅓ pound each)

Salt and pepper

Spray skillet with nonstick cooking spray and sauté mushrooms until tender. Add next three ingredients, combine, and simmer about 3 minutes. Season steaks with salt and pepper to taste. Brush marinade on steaks before and during cooking. Broil steaks for 10 to 15 minutes, or until flaky, turning once. Pour remaining marinade over steaks and serve.

Broiled Swordfish Steaks
with Salsa

serves **4**

I	15-ounce can black beans, rinsed and drained
1¼	cups frozen whole kernel corn, thawed
¾	cup purple onion, finely chopped
¾	cup sweet red pepper, finely chopped
2	jalapeño peppers, seeded and finely chopped
¼	cup balsamic vinegar
⅛	cup olive oil
1½	tablespoons Dijon mustard
¼	teaspoon salt
⅛	teaspoon pepper
	Nonstick cooking spray
4	swordfish steaks, 6–7 ounces each
2	tablespoons olive oil
¼	cup fresh cilantro, chopped

To make salsa: Combine first 10 ingredients; cover and chill for approximately 2 hours.

Preheat broiler. Spray broiler well with nonstick cooking spray. Brush steaks with 2 tablespoons oil and place on rack. Place rack approximately 6 inches from heat, broil steaks for 5 minutes. Baste, turn, baste again, and continue to broil for 5 to 8 minutes or until fish flakes easily with a fork.

Before serving, mix cilantro into black bean mixture. Serve over fish.

Note: You should limit your consumption of swordfish because of the elevated levels of mercury that can sometimes be associated with it. The FDA is currently creating guidelines for fish with elevated mercury content (these also include tuna and shark).

Salmon with Basil Pesto Marinade

serves **4**

2	cups fresh basil
2	tablespoons white pepper
I	lemon, juiced
2	tablespoons olive oil
2	large cloves garlic, chopped
	Nonstick cooking spray
4	boneless, skinless salmon fillets, 5–6 ounces each

In a blender, mix basil, pepper, lemon juice, olive oil, and garlic. Blend until a smooth paste has been formed. Coat a large baking dish evenly with nonstick cooking spray. Layer pan with fish fillets. Cover with half of pesto mixture. Place in preheated broiler. Cook for 5 minutes. Turn once and cover with remaining pesto marinade. Cook fish for additional 4 minutes or until fish flakes easily with a fork.

Chicken Entrées

Basic Marinated Chicken on the Grill

serves 4

This recipe is perfect for just about anything. Keep precooked chicken breasts in the refrigerator for salads, or add to pasta and rice dishes for a little extra protein.

2	tablespoons olive oil
I	tablespoon garlic, crushed
I	teaspoon each dried tarragon, basil, oregano, sage, and pepper
4	skinless, boneless chicken breasts

Heat outdoor grill to appropriate temperature. Mix olive oil and herbs until a paste is formed. Place breasts on grill and brush mixture on each breast. Cook 4 to 5 minutes on each side.

Chicken Florentine

	Nonstick cooking spray
½	cup onions, chopped
I	clove garlic, minced
½	cup mushrooms, chopped
I	8-ounce package frozen spinach, thawed, drained, and chopped
	Salt and pepper
½	cup part-skim ricotta cheese
4	skinless, boneless chicken breasts
½	cup white wine

Generously spray a large skillet with nonstick cooking spray. Add onions and garlic. Stir until onions are tender. Add mushrooms. Cook until browned, but tender. Remove from heat. Add spinach and salt and pepper. Cook for 2 to 3 minutes, until spinach is heated. Add cheese. Mix in mushrooms and remove from heat. In same pan, add chicken breasts. Add wine. Cook for 5 to 6 minutes on each side, or until chicken is done. Remove from pan. Place chicken in shallow baking dish sprayed with nonstick cooking spray. Top with mushroom and spinach mixture. Broil for 5 minutes.

120   The Everyday Meal Planner for Type 2 Diabetics

Chicken Cordon Bleu (Mock)

4   skinless, boneless chicken breasts
1   tablespoon olive oil
½   teaspoon garlic powder
¼   teaspoon fresh ground pepper
     Dash salt
     Nonstick cooking spray
2   ounces prosciutto ham
4   ounces Swiss cheese, shredded

Place chicken breasts between 2 sheets of waxed paper and press thin—about ¼ inch. In large skillet, heat oil over medium heat. Season with garlic powder, pepper, and salt. Sauté chicken on both sides for approximately 4 to 5 minutes. Remove chicken and place in shallow baking dish coated with nonstick cooking spray. Place ham and cheese over each chicken breast. Broil until cheese is melted and slightly browned.

Sweet and Sour
Chicken Skewers

serves 4

4   wooden skewers
¾   cup reduced-sugar or sugar-free apricot
      preserves
¼   cup white wine vinegar
1½   teaspoons hot pepper sauce
¾   pound chicken, boneless and skinless
1   sweet, red bell pepper, cut into 1-inch chunks
1   green bell pepper, cut into 1-inch chunks
1   small yellow onion, cut into 1-inch chunks
2   tablespoons olive oil
2   cups brown rice, cooked

Soak wooden skewers in water for 30 minutes (this prevents burning on the grill). Mix preserves and vinegar in a small saucepan over medium heat until blended. Add hot pepper sauce. Thread chicken, peppers, and onion onto skewers. Brush with sweet and sour mixture. Brush grill with olive oil and grill skewers for approximately 10 minutes, turning to even cooking. Chicken should appear white. Serve over brown rice.

Chicken Braised in Wine, with Mushrooms

serves 4

	Nonstick cooking spray
4	chicken breasts, skinned and deboned
¾	cup red wine
¾	cup mild onions, chopped
I	garlic clove, peeled and minced
2	tablespoons parsley, minced
I	bay leaf
½	teaspoon dried thyme
I	teaspoon salt
⅛	teaspoon pepper
½	pound sliced mushrooms

Spray a sauté pan or stockpot with nonstick cooking spray. Cook chicken breasts on each side until browned, about 5 to 7 minutes. Add wine and remaining ingredients, except the mushrooms. Simmer breasts in wine for about 10 minutes. Add mushrooms and simmer for 5 minutes more. Serve breasts with sauce ladled over them.

Turkey Entrées

Stuffed Green Peppers

serves 6

6	large green bell peppers
2	cups mushrooms, stalks removed and sliced thinly
I	small onion, chopped
	Nonstick cooking spray
I½	pounds lean ground turkey
I	clove garlic, minced
2	teaspoons dried basil
I	teaspoon dried oregano
I	teaspoon dried tarragon
	Salt and pepper
2	cups tomato juice

Wash and remove tops of peppers. Remove seeds and membrane. Set in large baking dish with ½ to I inch water at base. In large skillet, cook mushrooms and onions using nonstick cooking spray. Onions will appear translucent and mushrooms will be tender. Remove from heat. Cook turkey using nonstick cooking spray. Add garlic, basil, oregano, tarragon, and salt and pepper while cooking. Add cooked mushrooms, onion, and tomato juice to turkey meat. Add mixture to peppers. Cook peppers in oven at 375°F for 30 to 45 minutes. Peppers will be tender. As an alternative, try adding 2 cups of cooked brown rice to meat mixture before stuffing peppers.

Turkey Chili

2	tablespoons olive oil
I	clove garlic, minced
½	cup yellow onions, finely chopped
2	tablespoons green pepper, chopped
I	pound lean ground turkey
3	tablespoons yellow mustard
I	teaspoon salt
¼	teaspoon cayenne
3	tablespoons chili powder
2	tablespoons cumin
2	14-ounce cans tomatoes with juice
3–4	bay leaves
2	14-ounce cans kidney beans with juice

Heat olive oil in pan, and gently simmer garlic in the oil until liquefied but not brown. Add onions and green peppers, and sauté until tender. Add the ground turkey and stir until it is browned. Add mustard, salt, cayenne, chili powder, and cumin. Mix well and add the tomatoes with its juice. Lay bay leaves on top. Cover and simmer for 45 minutes. Add the beans with their liquid, stir, and cook uncovered for an additional 15 minutes.

Chili No. 2

I   small onion, chopped

I   clove garlic, minced

     Nonstick cooking spray

I ½   pounds lean ground turkey

I   12-ounce can tomato sauce

I   12-ounce can crushed tomatoes

I   can great Northern white beans, drained and rinsed

I   can pinto beans, drained and rinsed

I   can kidney beans, drained and rinsed

I   bag Carroll Shelby's Original Texas Brand Chili Kit (bag contains packet of masa flour for thickening; can be omitted)

In large skillet, sauté onion and garlic using nonstick cooking spray. Remove from heat. Add turkey and cook until browned. In large stockpot, add all remaining ingredients. Cook over medium heat until ingredients boil. Reduce heat to simmer and let cook for 45 minutes (this allows the flavors to blend and mature). (Serving size is I cup.)

Herbed Turkey, Wrapped in Foil or Cooked in Oven Bag

Roasting a turkey requires constant attention and basting. Cooking a turkey in foil, or in an oven bag, won't produce quite the same results as roasting, but it is far more convenient—saving time and effort.

1   turkey
    Olive oil
    Tarragon
    Rosemary
    Oregano
    Basil
    Sage
    Salt and pepper

Season the turkey well, inside and out, by rubbing it with olive oil and any or all of the remaining ingredients.

Wrap the bird in heavy duty aluminum foil, or use a Reynolds oven bag (read the directions on the box for the latter method). A 10- to 12-pound turkey needs to bake for between 3 ¼ to 3 ¾ hours at 325°F. Heavier birds will need approximately an additional 15 minutes per pound.

Other Entrées

Ham

If you choose to purchase an unbaked ham, and prepare it yourself, more power to you. If you purchase your ham "ready to eat" or "fully cooked," especially from a store that specializes in prepared hams, such as Honeybaked, just be careful of glazes that are usually high in sugar.

Preparing an unbaked ham: Preheat oven to 325°F. Place ham on rack in a shallow pan, uncovered. Whether it is a whole ham—typically 10 to 15 pounds, or half a ham—5 to 7 pounds—allow about 20 minutes cooking time per pound. A smaller ham may require cooking up to 35 minutes per pound. The internal temperature must be 160°F; use a meat thermometer to determine the temperature. Once the ham is cooked, remove the rind and all excess fat.

For a precooked ham, cooking time is slightly less; about 18 minutes per pound for a whole ham, and 18 to 24 minutes for a half ham per pound. The internal temperature should reach 140°F.

Savory Brisket

serves 10

Best done a day ahead.

2	large brown onions
5	pounds or more of fresh beef brisket (trim off as much fat as possible)
1	handful peppercorns
2	14-ounce cans stewed tomatoes
2	bay leaves
1	cup catsup or chili sauce
½	teaspoon kosher salt
½	cup dry red wine

Cut onions into ¼-inch rings and separate. Place one of the cut-up onions on the bottom of a roasting pan. Lay the brisket on top of the onions, work some of the peppercorns into the brisket, leaving the others scattered on top and around the meat. Pour the cans of stewed tomatoes over the meat. Add the remaining onions and bay leaves and cover with ketchup or chili sauce. Sprinkle with 2 to 3 pinches kosher salt. Finally, pour over the red wine. Cover tightly with foil and bake for 2½ hours at 325°F, or until fork enters the meat easily. Drain off liquid and separate fat from juice. Slice the brisket, and return to roasting pan. Either cover with onion and tomato drippings and juices, or blend onions and tomatoes in a food processor and cover sliced brisket with the juices and puree. Refrigerate overnight and reheat the next day for serving.

Beef Tenderloin with Pepper

serves 10 to 12

4   pounds fillet of beef
       Peppercorns, uncrushed
I   cup beef bouillon, prepared

Have your butcher remove all visible fat from the beef. Heat oven to
500°F. Roll over thin end of beef and tie with string. Roll beef in peppercorns. Using hands or spatula, press peppercorns into the beef.
Place the beef on a roasting pan rack so that the fat can run off.
Immediately reduce heat to 400°F and cook beef for 35 to 40 minutes. As beef cooks, continuously baste with beef bouillon, if necessary. Center of beef should read at least 130°F. Allow beef to sit for
15 minutes before cutting.

Side Dishes—Vegetables

Lightly Sautéed Spinach with Garlic

serves 4 to 6

2	large bunches spinach
I	tablespoon olive oil
5–6	garlic cloves, whole
	Cooking spray (olive oil)
	Pepper to taste
	Dash of salt

If spinach is unwashed, fill large sink with cold water and soak spinach, agitating water slightly to remove any sand. Remove stems and drain leaves. Do not pat dry. In large skillet, heat olive oil over medium heat. Add garlic cloves and simmer until brown and near tender; reduce heat if necessary to prevent cloves from burning. Place spinach in pan, and lightly spray it with olive oil cooking spray. Season with salt and pepper. Cover. Turn leaves periodically for even heat. Cook for 5 minutes.

Steamed Asparagus in Lemon Vinaigrette

serves 4 to 6

I   pound fresh asparagus
¼   cup fresh lemon juice
I   tablespoon olive oil
½   teaspoon salt
¼   teaspoon black pepper

Trim off the pithy ends of the asparagus. Steam asparagus for 10 to 12 minutes until tender but firm. Combine lemon juice, olive oil, salt, and pepper. Pour over asparagus while asparagus is still warm and serve.

Grilled Corn

serves 4

4   ears fresh corn, husked and cleaned
2   tablespoons olive oil
      Salt and pepper

Brush each ear lightly with olive oil. Season with salt and pepper. Wrap in foil, sealing edges. Cook on grill for 20 to 25 minutes, or until foil appears charred and corn is tender.

Ratatouille

1   tablespoon olive oil
2   cloves garlic, minced
1   cup onion, chopped
1   large eggplant, ¼ inch cubes, skin on
3   medium zucchini, ¼ inch cubes
2   medium yellow squash, ¼ inch cubes
1   red bell pepper, ¼ inch cubes
1   green bell pepper, ¼ inch cubes
2   cups mushrooms, sliced
5–6 Roma tomatoes, peeled, seeded, and chopped
1   tablespoon dried oregano
1   tablespoon dried basil
    Salt and pepper

Heat oil in large skillet. Add garlic and onions and cook until tender. Add all vegetables and stir well. Let simmer for about 5 minutes. Add herbs and salt and pepper and cook a few minutes more. (Serving size is ½ cup.)

Steamed Broccoli Florets

serves 2 to 4

Visualize one floret of broccoli that is roughly the size of a lightbulb. That represents roughly 1 cup of broccoli, which is 2 servings of vegetables.

	Water
1	bunch broccoli
1	teaspoon lemon juice
2	tablespoons nonfat sour cream
1	sprinkle Butter Buds or Molly McButter
1	tablespoon almond slivers

In large steaming pot, bring water to a boil. As water comes to a boil, thoroughly wash broccoli and trim ends. Place broccoli in pot. Cover and steam for 10 to 12 minutes.

For sauce: Add 1 teaspoon lemon juice to 2 tablespoons nonfat sour cream, or add a sprinkle of Butter Buds or Molly McButter with 1 tablespoon almond slivers.

Green Beans, Steamed

Steaming vegetables instead of boiling them preserves many of their nutrients and their color. Steamed green beans are a quick, easy, and nutritious addition to fish, ham, or any number of dishes.

Water
Green beans
Butter Buds
Lemon juice

Wash green beans and break off their ends. Use a steamer (a cooking pot with a colander that fits down into it); fill pot with water to below bottom of colander. Bring water to a boil, put in green beans, and cover. Cooking time will be between 15 and 20 minutes. Remove colander, drain beans, transfer them into a serving dish; sprinkle with Butter Buds, and squeeze a little lemon juice over them, if desired.

Roasted Portobello Mushrooms

serves **4**

2   garlic cloves, chopped
     Nonstick cooking spray
4   large Portobello mushrooms
2   tablespoons olive oil
     Pepper
½   cup white wine

In small pan, cook garlic until brown using nonstick cooking spray. Wash mushrooms and remove stems. Use nonstick cooking spray on large baking dish. Place mushrooms cap side down. Place garlic in each mushroom. Brush with olive oil (or use cooking spray to save 60 calories). Sprinkle with pepper. Place in 400°F oven. Cook for 10 minutes, then baste each mushroom with wine. Bake for 20 minutes or until Portobello mushrooms cut easily and appear tender.

Grilled Artichokes with Cilantro Pesto

serves 4 to 8

1	tablespoon lemon juice
¼–½	teaspoon salt
3	cloves garlic, sliced
4	artichokes, bottoms cut flush and leaves snipped
2	teaspoons olive oil
1	recipe of cilantro pesto

Combine lemon juice, salt, and garlic in a small stockpot. Add artichokes and simmer in about 2 inches of water for 20 to 30 minutes or until just tender. Set aside or refrigerate for later use. When ready to grill, halve the artichokes and brush with olive oil. Cook on a well-oiled rack over a medium-hot fire for 10 to 12 minutes, grilling cut side first. Flip to heat the outer edges briefly. Serve with Cilantro Pesto.

Cilantro Pesto*

2	tablespoons pistachio nuts, shelled
¼	cup water
2	tablespoons olive oil
½	teaspoon sea salt
2	cloves garlic
1	cup cilantro leaves

Blend all ingredients until smooth. Serve with grilled artichokes.

*Printed with permission by McGraw-Hill. Patti A. Bess, Vegetarian Barbecue & Other Pleasures of the Harvest, 1999, pp. 109, 115.

Side Dishes— Grains, Beans, and Other Starches

Brown Rice with Herbs and Mushrooms

serves 4

2½   cups beef broth
1   cup brown rice
2   cups sliced mushrooms
¼   cup parsley, finely chopped

Bring broth to boil in a large pan. Add rice, mushrooms, and parsley. Stir. Reduce heat to simmer. Cover and cook for 20 minutes. Remove from heat and fluff with fork.

Bulgur Pilaf

½   cup onion, diced
1   tablespoon olive oil
1   cup bulgur
½   cup celery, chopped
2   cups broth, vegetable or chicken
½   teaspoon dried marjoram
¼   teaspoon sage
    Salt and pepper

Sauté onions with oil in large skillet until translucent. Add bulgur, celery, and broth. Add marjoram, sage, and salt and pepper. Bring to a boil. Reduce heat and simmer, covered, for approximately 35 to 40 minutes. Bulgur will appear fluffy.

Mashed Sweet Potatoes

serves *4*

5	medium sweet potatoes
2	tablespoons Butter Buds
¼	cup nonfat milk
2–3	tablespoons orange rind zest
I	tablespoon ground cinnamon
½	tablespoon ground cloves

Place potatoes in boiling water. Cover and cook for 25 minutes. Peel skin and mash in large bowl. Add Butter Buds. Warm milk in microwave. Add a tablespoon at a time to acquire favored consistency of potatoes. Add orange zest, cinnamon, and cloves.

Oven-Roasted New Potatoes

serves *6 to 7*

12–15	small red or new potatoes (about I½ pounds)
2	tablespoons olive oil
4	cloves garlic, minced
2	tablespoons fresh rosemary, finely chopped
	Pepper

Scrub potatoes and dry thoroughly with paper towel. Rub evenly with olive oil and roll in garlic, rosemary, and pepper. Place potatoes on baking sheet. Bake at 400°F for 40 minutes or until tender.

Deviled Eggs Light

serves 12

12 eggs
    Nonfat mayonnaise
2   tablespoons dry mustard
    Worcestershire sauce
    Salt and pepper
    Paprika

In large pot, place eggs in cold water. Bring water to a boil. Reduce heat to simmer. Cook for 12 minutes. Once finished, place eggs in cold water. De-shell eggs and cut lengthwise. Place yolks in small bowl. Add nonfat mayonnaise to desired consistency. Add 2 tablespoons to begin, then gradually add more if needed. Egg yolks should be creamy in texture. Add dry mustard, a dash of Worcestershire sauce, and salt and pepper. Sprinkle with paprika. Chill for 30 minutes before serving. Stuff whites with mixture.

Fettuccine and Spinach

serves 6

½ package fettuccine (total of ½ pound dry
    weight)
2   tablespoons olive oil
2   cloves garlic, crushed
1   10-ounce package frozen chopped spinach,
    thawed and drained
1   cup nonfat ricotta cheese
¼   cup fresh parsley, chopped
1   teaspoon dried basil
    Salt and pepper
2–3 tablespoons Parmesan cheese, grated

Cook pasta according to instructions. In separate pan, sauté spinach
and garlic in oil. Add cheese, parsley, basil, and salt and pepper. Toss
with noodles. Sprinkle with Parmesan cheese.

Desserts

Angel Food Cake with Fresh Fruit

serves 10 to 12

2   large peaches, peeled and sliced
2   cups strawberries, sliced
1½   cups blueberries
1   small banana, sliced
1   lemon
1   angel food cake, store bought*

In large bowl, mix peaches, strawberries, blueberries, and banana. Squeeze juice of lemon over the fruit. On individual plates, place 1 slice of cake (1 ounce or ½2 cake). Top with ½ cup fruit.

Sponge cake offers a lower glycemic value and can be used as a substitution.

Fruit Kabobs

serves 8

2   large apples (any variety)
2   large peaches, firm
3   cups strawberries
2   cups grapes
8   wooden skewers

Cut apples and peaches into 1-inch cubes. Wash and trim strawberries. Cut berries in half. Rinse grapes. Rinse skewers in cold water, and thread fruit onto each skewer.

Red, White, and Blue Parfaits

serves 4

2   cups fresh blueberries
I   tablespoon lemon juice
I   small package fat-free, sugar-free vanilla pudding
2   cups sliced strawberries, fresh or frozen without sugar
½   cup whipped cream (low fat, low sugar)

Blend blueberries in food processor; add lemon juice and set aside. Prepare pudding according to package directions. Place ⅛ pudding mixture into each of four small parfait glass, then layer with ⅛ of blueberry puree. Layer the rest of the pudding in the glasses, then top with strawberries and whipped cream.

Chocolate Cheesecake*

serves 12

	Nonstick vegetable cooking spray
2	cups nonfat cottage cheese
2	eggs
⅓	cup sugar
	Acesulfame K sugar substitute equivalent to ⅓ cup sugar
4	ounces Neufchatel cheese, softened
⅓	cup cocoa
I	teaspoon vanilla extract

Preheat oven to 300°F. Coat an 8¼-by-12¼ inch pan or a 9-inch springform pan with nonstick cooking spray. In a large bowl, using an electric mixer, blend the cottage cheese, eggs, sugar, sugar substitute, Neufchatel cheese, cocoa, and vanilla extract until smooth. Pour into the prepared pan. Bake for 35 minutes, or until edges are set. Cool completely on a wire rack. Refrigerate for 4 hours, or until thoroughly chilled, before serving.

*Reprinted with permission by McGraw-Hill. Lois M. Soneral, The Type 2 Diabetes Desserts Cookboook, 1999, p. 48.

Pumpkin Chiffon Pie*

serves 8

I	ounce instant sugar-free vanilla pudding
½	teaspoon cinnamon
¼	teaspoon ground ginger
½	teaspoon nutmeg
I	15-ounce can, solid pack pumpkin
½	cup 2% milk
⅛	cup water
2	egg whites
⅛	cup sugar
2	packets Acesulfame K sugar substitute
I	8-inch prepared graham cracker or shortbread pie crust
½	cup nonfat whipped topping

In a large bowl, using an electric mixer on low speed, blend the pudding mix, spices, pumpkin, milk, and water for 3 to 4 minutes until well combined. In a medium bowl, beat the egg whites until frothy. Gradually add the sugar and sugar substitute to the egg whites, beating constantly, until soft peaks form. Fold in the pudding mixture. Pour into the prepared crust. Refrigerate for 4 hours. Top each serving with I tablespoon of the whipped topping.

*Reprinted with permission by McGraw-Hill. Lois M. Soneral, The Type 2 Diabetes Desserts Cookboook, *1999, p. 64.*

Vanilla Ice Milk
with Baked Pears

serves **4**

2   large pears, peeled and cored

2   tablespoons water

1   ounce walnuts, finely chopped

1   teaspoon lemon juice

1   tablespoon cinnamon

½   cup sugar-free cream soda

2   cups vanilla ice milk

Preheat oven to 350°F degrees. In deep baking dish, position pears in 2 tablespoons water. Sprinkle pears with nuts, lemon juice, and cinnamon. Place in oven and bake for 30 minutes, basting with sugar-free cream soda. Remove from oven and slice each pear into 4 pieces. In each dish, place ½ cup vanilla ice milk. Cover with pear slices.

Note that cooking fruit may alter the rate at which blood sugar rises as it is absorbed. If this presents a concern, please opt for raw fruit. This dessert is lovely with fresh, uncooked pears and a dash of cinnamon.

Fruit-Topped, Low-Fat Lemon Cheesecake*

serves 10

Nonstick vegetable cooking spray
¼ cup graham cracker crumbs
8 ounces nonfat cream cheese
1 14-ounce can nonfat, sweetened, condensed milk
3 egg whites
1 whole egg
⅓ cup lemon juice concentrate, thawed
1 teaspoon vanilla extract
¼ cup all-purpose flour
1 cup seasonal fresh fruit

Preheat oven to 300°F. Coat the bottom of an angel food cake pan with nonstick cooking spray. Sprinkle the graham cracker crumbs evenly on the bottom of the pan. In a large bowl using the electric mixer, beat the cream cheese until fluffy. Gradually add the condensed milk and beat until smooth. Add the egg whites, whole egg, lemon juice concentrate, and vanilla extract. Stir in the flour. Blend well. Pour into the prepared pan. Bake for 45 to 50 minutes, or until a tester inserted in the center comes out clean. Cool. Refrigerate for 3 to 4 hours. Top with fresh fruit before serving.

*Reprinted with permission by McGraw-Hill. Lois M. Soneral, The Type 2 Diabetes Desserts Cookboook, *1999, p. 64.*

APPENDIX

Food Composition Tables

All units of carbohydrates and protein are expressed in grams.

Name	Amount	Calories	Carbohydrate	Protein
Beverages				
Beer, light	12 fl oz	95	5	1
Beer, regular	12 fl oz	150	13	1
Club Soda	12 fl oz	0	0	0
Coffee, brewed	4 fl oz	0	0	0
Coffee, instant, prepared	4 fl oz	0	1	0
Cola, diet, aspartame or saccharin	12 fl oz	0	0	0
Cola, regular	12 fl oz	160	41	0
Fruit punch drink, canned	4 fl oz	57	14	0
Gin, rum, vodka, whisky 80-proof	1.5 fl oz	95	0	0
Ginger ale	12 fl oz	125	32	0
Grape drink, canned	4 fl oz	68	17	0
Grape soda	12 fl oz	180	46	0
Lemon-lime soda	12 fl oz	155	39	0
Lemonade, concentrate, frozen, diluted	4 fl oz	56	14	0
Orange soda	12 fl oz	180	46	0

Name	Amount	Calories	Carbohydrate	Protein
Root beer	12 fl oz	165	42	0
Tea, brewed	4 fl oz	0	0	0
Tea, instant, prepared, sweetened	4 fl oz	44	11	0
Tea, instant, prepared, unsweetened	4 fl oz	0	0	0
Wine, dessert	3.5 fl oz	140	8	0
Wine, table, red	3.5 fl oz	75	3	0
Wine, table, white	3.5 fl oz	80	3	0

Cheese

Name	Amount	Calories	Carbohydrate	Protein
Blue cheese	1 oz	100	1	6
Camembert cheese	1 wedge	115	0	8
Cheddar cheese	1 oz	115	0	7
Cheddar cheese, shredded	1 cup	455	1	28
Cottage cheese, creamed, small curd	1 cup	215	6	26
Cottage cheese, creamed, with fruit	1 cup	280	30	22
Cottage cheese, low fat 2%	1 cup	205	8	31
Cream cheese	1 oz	100	1	2
Feta cheese	1 oz	75	1	4
Mozzarella cheese, skim, low moisture	1 oz	80	1	8
Muenster cheese	1 oz	105	0	7
Parmesan cheese, grated	1 tbsp	25	0	2
	1 oz	130	1	12
Provolone cheese	1 oz	100	1	7
Ricotta cheese, whole milk	1 cup	430	7	28
Ricotta cheese, part skim milk	1 cup	340	13	28
	1 oz	85	3	7

Name	Amount	Calories	Carbohydrate	Protein
Swiss cheese	1 oz	105	1	8
Pasteurized process cheese, American	1 oz	105	0	6
Pasteurized process cheese, Swiss	1 oz	95	1	7
Pasteurized process cheese food, American	1 oz	95	2	6
Pasteurized process cheese spread, American	1 oz	80	2	5

Dairy Products

Name	Amount	Calories	Carbohydrate	Protein
Buttermilk, dried	1 cup	465	59	41
Buttermilk, fluid	1 cup	100	12	8
Chocolate milk, low fat 1%	1 cup	160	26	8
Chocolate milk, regular	1 cup	210	26	8
Cocoa powder with nonfat dry milk, prepared	1 serv	100	22	3
Cocoa powder without nonfat dry milk, prepared	1 serv	225	30	9
Eggnog	1 cup	340	34	10
Evaporated milk, skim, canned	1 cup	200	29	19
Half and half, cream	1 tbsp	20	1	0
Ice cream, vanilla, regular 11% fat	1 cup	270	32	5
Ice cream, vanilla, rich 16% fat	1 cup	350	32	4
Ice cream, vanilla, soft serve	1 cup	375	38	7
Ice milk, vanilla, soft serve 3% fat	1 cup	225	38	8
Imitation sour cream dressing	1 tbsp	20	1	0
Imitation whipped topping, pressurized	1 tbsp	10	1	0

Name	Amount	Calories	Carbohydrate	Protein
Light, coffee or table cream	1 tbsp	30	1	0
Milk, low fat, 1%, no added solids	1 cup	100	12	8
Milk, low fat, 2%, no added solids	1 cup	120	12	8
Milk, skim, no added solids	1 cup	85	12	8
Nonfat dry milk, instant	1 cup	245	35	24
Sherbet, 2% fat	1 cup	270	59	2
Sour cream	1 tbsp	10	0	0
Whipping cream, unwhipped, light	1 tbsp	45	0	0
Whipped topping, pressurized	1/2 cup	78	4	1
	1 tbsp	10	0	0
Yogurt, with low fat milk, fruit flavored	1 cup	230	43	10
Yogurt, with low fat milk, plain	1 cup	145	16	12
Yogurt, with nonfat milk, plain	1 cup	125	17	13

Dressings

Name	Amount	Calories	Carbohydrate	Protein
Blue cheese salad dressing	1 tbsp	75	1	1
French salad dressing, regular	1 tbsp	85	1	0
French salad dressing, low calorie	1 tbsp	25	2	0
Italian salad dressing, regular	1 tbsp	80	1	0
Italian salad dressing, low calorie	1 tbsp	5	2	0
Mayonnaise, regular	1 tbsp	100	0	0

Name	Amount	Calories	Carbohydrate	Protein
Mayonnaise, imitation	1 tbsp	35	2	0
Mayonnaise type salad dressing	1 tbsp	60	4	0
Tartar sauce	1 tbsp	75	1	0
1000 Island salad dressing, regular	1 tbsp	60	2	0
1000 Island salad dressing, low calorie	1 tbsp	25	2	0
Vinegar and oil salad dressing	1 tbsp	70	0	0

Eggs

Name	Amount	Calories	Carbohydrate	Protein
Eggs, raw, white	1	15	0	4
Eggs, raw, whole	1	75	1	6

Fats

Name	Amount	Calories	Carbohydrate	Protein
Butter, salted	1 tbsp	100	0	0
Butter, unsalted	1 tbsp	100	0	0
Fats, cooking/vegetable shortening	1 tbsp	115	0	0
Lard	1 tbsp	115	0	0
Margarine, regular, hard, 80% fat	1 tbsp	35	0	0
Margarine, regular, soft, 80% fat	1 tbsp	75	0	0
Corn oil	1 tbsp	125	0	0
Olive oil	1 tbsp	125	0	0
Peanut oil	1 tbsp	125	0	0
Safflower oil	1 tbsp	125	0	0
Soybean oil, hydrogenated	1 tbsp	125	0	0
Soybean-cottonseed oil, hydrogenated	1 tbsp	125	0	0
Sunflower oil	1 tbsp	125	0	0

Name	Amount	Calories	Carbohydrate	Protein

Fish and Shellfish

Name	Amount	Calories	Carbohydrate	Protein
Clams, raw	3 oz	65	2	11
Clams, canned, drained	3 oz	85	2	13
Crabmeat, canned	1 cup	135	1	23
Crabmeat, steamed	3 oz	80	0	15
Fish sticks, frozen, reheated	1	70	4	6
Flounder or sole, baked, with butter	3 oz	120	0	16
Flounder or sole, baked, without fat	3 oz	80	0	17
Haddock, breaded, fried	3 oz	175	7	17
Halibut, broiled, butter, with lemon juice	3 oz	140	0	20
Halibut, Atlantic/Pacific, meat only, raw	3 oz	114	0	24
Herring, pickled	3 oz	190	0	17
Oysters, raw	1 cup	160	8	20
Oysters, breaded, fried	1	90	5	5
Salmon, canned, pink, with bones	3 oz	120	0	17
Salmon, baked, red	3 oz	140	0	21
Salmon, smoked	3 oz	150	0	18
Sardines, Atlantic, canned, with oil, drained	3 oz	175	0	20
Sea bass, white, flesh only, raw	3 oz	82	0	18
Scallops, raw	3 oz	69	3	13
Shrimp, canned, drained	3 oz	100	1	21
Shrimp, French fried	3 oz	200	11	16
Trout, broiled, with butter and lemon juice	3 oz	175	0	21
Trout, brook, flesh only	3 oz	86	0	16
Tuna, canned, drained, oil, chunk, light	3 oz	165	0	24

Name	Amount	Calories	Carbohydrate	Protein
Tuna, canned,				
drained, water, white	3 oz	135	0	30
Tuna salad	1 cup	375	19	33

Fruit

Name	Amount	Calories	Carbohydrate	Protein
Apples, raw, unpeeled,				
3 per lb.	1	80	21	0
Apples, raw, peeled, sliced	1 cup	65	16	0
Apples, dried, sulfured	10 rings	155	42	1
Apple juice, canned	1 cup	115	29	0
Applesauce, canned,				
unsweetened	1 cup	105	28	0
Apricots, raw	3	50	12	1
Apricots, canned,				
heavy syrup	3 halves	70	18	0
Apricots, canned,				
juice pack	1 cup	120	31	2
	3 halves	40	10	1
Apricots, dried, cooked,				
unsweetened	1 cup	210	55	3
Apricot nectar,				
no added vitamin C	1 cup	140	36	1
Avocados, California	1	305	12	4
Avocados, Florida	1	340	27	5
Bananas	1	105	27	1
Bananas, sliced	1 cup	140	35	2
Blackberries, raw	1 cup	75	18	1
Blueberries, raw	1 cup	80	20	1
Blueberries, frozen,				
sweetened	1 cup	185	50	1
Cherries, sour, red,				
canned, water	1 cup	90	22	2
Cherries, sweet, raw	10	50	11	1
Cranberry juice cocktail				
with vitamin C	1 cup	145	38	0

Name	Amount	Calories	Carbohydrate	Protein
Cranberry sauce, canned, sweetened	1 cup	420	108	1
Dates	10	230	61	2
Figs, dried	10	475	122	6
Fruit cocktail, canned, juice pack	1 cup	115	29	1
Grapefruit, raw, pink, white	½	40	10	1
Grapefruit, canned, syrup pack	1 cup	150	39	1
Grapefruit juice, raw	1 cup	95	23	1
Grapes, European, raw, Thompson	10	35	9	0
Grape juice, canned	1 cup	155	38	1
Grape juice, frozen, diluted, sweetened, with vitamin C	1 cup	125	32	0
Kiwi, raw	1	45	11	1
Lemons/limes, raw	1	15	5	1
Lemon/lime juice, canned	1 tbsp	5	1	0
Mango, raw	1	135	35	1
Cantaloupe, raw	½	95	22	2
Honeydew melon, raw	1/10	45	12	1
Nectarine, raw	1	65	16	1
Orange, raw	1	60	15	1
Orange juice, chilled	1 cup	110	25	2
Papaya, raw	1 cup	65	17	1
Peach, raw	1	35	10	1
Peaches, canned, juice pack	1 cup	110	29	2
Pears, raw, Bartlett	1	100	25	1
Pears, canned, juice pack	1 cup	125	32	1
Pineapple, raw, diced	1 cup	75	19	1
Pineapple, canned, juice pack	1 cup	150	39	1
Plums, raw, 2⅛-inch diameter	1	35	9	1

Name	Amount	Calories	Carbohydrate	Protein
Plums, canned, juice pack	3	55	14	0
Prunes, dried	5 large	115	31	1
Prunes, dried, cooked, unsweetened	1 cup	225	60	2
Prune juice, canned	1 cup	180	45	2
Raisins	1 cup	435	115	5
	1 pkt	40	11	0
Raspberries, raw	1 cup	60	14	1
Rhubarb, cooked, added sugar	1 cup	280	75	1
Strawberries, raw	1 cup	45	10	1
Strawberries, frozen, sweetened	1 cup	245	66	1
Tangerine, raw	1	35	9	1
Watermelon, raw	1 pc	155	35	3
Watermelon, raw, diced	1 cup	50	11	1

Grains/Starches

Breads, Cereals, Cakes, Pasta, Rice, etc.

Name	Amount	Calories	Carbohydrate	Protein
Bagels, plain	1	200	38	7
Baking powder biscuits, from mix	1 biscuit	95	14	2
Bread crumbs, dry, grated	1 cup	390	73	13
Bread stuffing, from mix, moist	1 cup	420	40	9
Buckwheat flour, light, sifted	1 cup	340	78	6
Cornmeal, degerminated, enriched, cooked	1 cup	120	26	3
Cracked wheat bread	1 slice	65	12	2
French bread	1 slice	100	18	3
Italian bread	1 slice	85	17	3
Mixed grain bread	1 slice	65	12	2
Oatmeal bread	1 slice	65	12	2
Pita bread	1	165	33	6
Pumpernickel bread	1 slice	80	16	3

Name	Amount	Calories	Carbohydrate	Protein
Raisin bread	1 slice	65	13	2
Rolls, dinner, from mix	1	85	14	2
Rolls, frankfurter or hamburger	1	115	20	3
Rolls, hard	1	155	30	5
Rolls, hoagie or submarine	1	400	72	11
Rye bread, light	1 slice	65	12	2
Tortillas, corn	1	65	13	2
Vienna bread	1 slice	70	13	2
Wheat bread	1 slice	65	12	2
Wheat bread, toasted	1 slice	65	12	3
Wheat flour, all purpose, sifted	1 cup	420	88	12
Whole wheat bread	1 slice	70	13	3
Corn grits, cooked, regular, yellow, no salt	1 cup	145	31	3
Cream of Wheat, cooked, regular, instant, no salt	1 cup	140	29	4
Malt-O-Meal, without salt	1 cup	120	26	4
Oatmeal, cooked, instant, plain, fortified	1 pkt	105	18	4
Oatmeal, cooked, regular, quick, instant, without salt	1 cup	145	25	6
All-Bran cereal	1 oz	70	21	4
Cheerios cereal	1 oz	110	20	4
Corn Flakes, Kellogg's	1 oz	110	24	2
40% Bran Flakes, Post	1 oz	90	22	3
Golden Grahams cereal	1 oz	110	24	2
Grape-Nuts cereal	1 oz	100	23	3
Nature Valley granola cereal	1 oz	125	19	3
Product 19 cereal	1 oz	110	24	3
Raisin Bran, Post	1 oz	85	21	3
Rice Krispies cereal	1 oz	110	25	2
Shredded Wheat cereal	1 oz	100	23	3
Special K cereal	1 oz	110	21	6

Name	Amount	Calories	Carbohydrate	Protein
Total cereal	1 oz	100	22	3
Wheaties cereal	1 oz	100	23	3
Angel food cake, from mix	1 pc	125	29	3
Carrot cake, with cream cheese frosting, from home recipe	1 pc	385	48	4
Cheesecake	1 pc	280	26	5
Coffee cake, crumb, from mix	1 pc	230	38	5
Devil's food cake, with chocolate frosting, from mix	1 pc	235	40	3
	1 cupcake	120	20	2
Fruitcake, dark, from home recipe	1 pc	165	25	2
Gingerbread cake, from mix	1 pc	175	32	2
Pound cake, from home recipe	1 loaf	2,025	265	33
	1 slice	120	15	2
Pound cake, from mix	1 slice	110	15	2
Sheetcake, with white frosting, from home recipe	1 pc	445	77	4
White cake, with white frosting, from mix	1 pc	260	42	3
Yellow cake, with chocolate frosting, from mix	1 pc	245	39	2
Brownies with nuts, frosting, commercial	1	100	16	1
Chocolate chip cookies, from mix	4	180	28	2
Chocolate chip cookies, from refrigerated dough	4	225	32	2
Fig bars	4	210	42	2
Oatmeal cookies, with raisins	4	245	36	3

Name	Amount	Calories	Carbohydrate	Protein
Peanut butter cookies, from home recipe	4	245	28	4
Sandwich type cookies	4	195	29	2
Sugar cookies, from refrigerated dough	4	235	31	2
Cheese crackers, plain	10	50	6	1
Cheese crackers, sandwich, with peanut butter	1	40	5	1
Graham crackers, plain	2	60	11	1
Melba toast, plain	1 pc	20	4	1
Rye wafers, whole grain	2	55	10	1
Saltine crackers	4	50	9	1
Snack type crackers	1	15	2	0
Wheat, thin crackers	4	35	5	1
Whole wheat wafers, crackers	2	35	5	1
Blueberry muffins, from mix	1	140	22	3
Bran muffins, from mix	1	140	24	3
Corn muffins, from mix	1	145	22	3
Croissants	1	235	27	5
Danish pastry, plain, no nuts	1	220	26	4
	1 oz	110	13	2
Danish pastry, with fruit	1	235	28	4
Doughnuts, cake type, plain	1	210	24	3
Doughnuts, yeast-leavened, glazed	1	235	26	4
English muffins, plain	1	140	27	5
French toast, from home recipe	1 slice	155	17	6
Pancakes, plain, from mix	1	60	8	2
Waffles, from mix	1	205	27	7
Apple pie	1 pc	405	60	3
Blueberry pie	1 pc	380	55	4
Cherry pie	1 pc	410	61	4
Cream Pie	1 pc	455	59	3
Pecan pie	1 pc	575	71	7

Name	Amount	Calories	Carbohydrate	Protein
Pumpkin pie	1 pc	320	37	6
Corn chips	1 oz	155	16	2
Popcorn, air-popped, unsalted	1 cup	30	6	1
Popcorn, popped, vegetable oil, salted	1 cup	55	6	1
Pretzels, stick	10	10	2	0
Macaroni, cooked, tender, hot	1 cup	155	32	5
Noodles, egg, cooked	1 cup	200	37	7
Noodles, chow mein, canned	1 cup	220	26	6
Rice, brown, cooked	1 cup	230	50	5
Rice, white, cooked	1 cup	225	50	4
Spaghetti, cooked, tender	1 cup	155	32	5
Beans, Peas, Legumes				
Black beans, dry, cooked, drained	1 cup	225	41	15
Black-eyed peas, dry, cooked	1 cup	190	35	13
Lentils, dry, cooked	1 cup	180	4	4
Lima beans, baby, frozen, cooked, drained	1 cup	190	35	12
Pea beans, dry, cooked, drained	1 cup	225	40	15
Peas, split, dry, cooked	1 cup	230	42	16
Pinto beans, dry, cooked, drained	1 cup	265	49	15
Red kidney beans, dry, canned	1 cup	230	42	15

Meat

Name	Amount	Calories	Carbohydrate	Protein
Beef, canned, corned	3 oz	185	0	22
Beef, cooked, bottom round, lean with fat	3 oz	220	0	25

Name	Amount	Calories	Carbohydrate	Protein
Beef, cooked, bottom round, lean only	2.8 oz	175	0	25
Beef, cooked, chuck blade, lean with fat	3 oz	325	0	22
Ground beef, broiled, lean	3 oz	230	0	21
Ground beef, broiled, regular	3 oz	245	0	20
Beef roast, rib, lean only	2.2 oz	150	0	17
Beef roast, rib, lean with fat	3 oz	315	0	19
Beef roast, round eye, lean	2.6 oz	135	0	22
Beef roast, round eye, lean with fat	3 oz	205	0	23
Beef steak, sirloin, broiled, lean with fat	3 oz	240	0	23
Beef steak, sirloin, broiled, lean only	2.5 oz	150	0	22
Lamb, chops, loin, broiled, lean only	2.3 oz	140	0	19
Lamb, chops, loin, broiled, lean with fat	2.8 oz	235	0	22
Lamb, leg, roasted, lean only	2.6 oz	140	0	20
Lamb, rib, roasted, lean only	2 oz	130	0	15
Pork, cured, bacon, regular, cooked	3 slices	110	0	6
Pork, cured, ham, roasted, lean	2.4 oz	105	0	17
Pork, luncheon meat, cooked ham, regular	2 slices	105	2	10
Pork, luncheon meat, cooked ham, lean	2 slices	75	1	11
Pork chop, loin, broiled, lean	2.5 oz	165	0	23
Pork chop, loin, pan fried, lean	2.4 oz	180	0	19

Name	Amount	Calories	Carbohydrate	Protein
Veal cutlet, medium fat, braised, broiled	3 oz	185	0	23

Meat Products

Name	Amount	Calories	Carbohydrate	Protein
Bologna	2 slices	180	2	7
Brown and serve sausage, browned	1 link	50	0	2
Frankfurter, cooked	1	145	1	5
Salami, dry type	2 slices	85	1	5

Meals/Prepared Recipes

Name	Amount	Calories	Carbohydrate	Protein
Beef and vegetable stew, from home recipe	1 cup	220	15	16
Cheeseburger, regular	1	300	28	15
Chicken à la king, from home recipe	1 cup	470	12	27
Chicken chow mein, canned	1 cup	95	18	7
Chicken pot pie, from from home recipe	1 pc	545	42	23
Chili con carne, with beans, canned	1 cup	340	31	19
Spaghetti, meatballs, tomato sauce, from home recipe	1 cup	330	39	19
Spaghetti, tomato sauce with cheese, from home recipe	1 cup	260	37	9
Enchilada	1	235	24	20
English muffin, egg, cheese, bacon	1	360	31	18
Fish sandwich, regular, with cheese	1	420	39	16
Hamburger, 4 oz patty	1	245	28	12
Macaroni and cheese, canned	1 cup	230	26	9
Quiche Lorraine	1 slice	600	29	13

Name	Amount	Calories	Carbohydrate	Protein
Pizza, cheese	1 slice	445	38	25
Roast beef sandwich	1	290	39	15
Taco	1	345	34	22

Nuts and Seeds

Name	Amount	Calories	Carbohydrate	Protein
Almonds, slivered	1 cup	795	28	27
Almonds, whole	1 oz	165	6	6
Brazil nuts	1 oz	185	4	4
Cashew nuts, dry roasted, unsalted	1 oz	165	9	4
Filberts (hazelnuts), chopped	1 oz	180	4	4
Macadamia nuts, oil roasted, salted	1 oz	205	4	2
Mixed nuts with peanuts, oil, unsalted	1 oz	175	6	5
Peanuts, oil roasted, salted	1 oz	165	5	8
Peanut butter	1 tbsp	95	3	5
Pine nuts	1 oz	160	5	3
Pistachio nuts	1 oz	165	7	6
Sesame seeds	1 tbsp	45	1	2
Sunflower seeds	1 oz	160	5	6
Walnuts, English, pieces	1 oz	180	5	4

Poultry

Name	Amount	Calories	Carbohydrate	Protein
Chicken, canned, boneless	5 oz	235	0	31
Chicken, roasted, breast	3 oz	140	0	27
Chicken, roasted, drumstick	1.6 oz	75	0	12
Chicken frankfurter	1	115	3	6
Duck, roasted, flesh only	½	445	0	52
Turkey, roasted, dark meat	4 pcs	160	0	24
Turkey, roasted, light meat	2 pcs	135	0	25

Sauces

Name	Amount	Calories	Carbohydrate	Protein
Barbecue sauce	1 tbsp	10	2	0
Beef gravy, canned	½ cup	65	6	4

Name	Amount	Calories	Carbohydrate	Protein
Cheese sauce with milk, from mix	½ cup	153	13	8
Chicken gravy, canned	½ cup	98	7	2
Hollandaise sauce with water, from mix	½ cup	120	7	3
Soy sauce	1 tbsp	10	2	2
White sauce with milk, from mix	½ cup	120	10	5

Soups

Name	Amount	Calories	Carbohydrate	Protein
Bean with bacon soup, canned	1 cup	170	23	8
Beef broth, bouillon, consommé, canned	1 cup	15	0	3
Chicken noodle soup, canned	1 cup	75	9	4
Chicken noodle soup, dehydrated, prepared	1 pkt	40	6	2
Clam chowder, Manhattan, canned	1 cup	80	12	4
Clam chowder, New England, with milk	1 cup	165	17	9
Minestrone soup, canned	1 cup	80	11	4
Onion soup, dehydrated, prepared	1 pkt	20	4	1
Pea soup, green, canned	1 cup	165	27	9
Tomato soup with milk, canned	1 cup	160	22	6
Tomato soup with water, canned	1 cup	85	17	2
Vegetable beef soup, canned	1 cup	80	10	6
Vegetarian soup, canned	1 cup	70	12	2

Name	Amount	Calories	Carbohydrate	Protein

Soy Foods

Name	Amount	Calories	Carbohydrate	Protein
Miso	1 cup	470	65	29
Soybeans, dry, cooked, drained	1 cup	235	19	20
Tofu	1 pc	85	3	9

Sweets

Candy, Desserts, Sugar

Name	Amount	Calories	Carbohydrate	Protein
Caramels, plain or chocolate	1 oz	115	22	1
Fudge, chocolate, plain	1 oz	115	21	1
Gumdrops	1 oz	100	25	0
Hard candy	1 oz	110	28	0
Jelly beans	1 oz	105	26	0
Marshmallows	1 oz	90	23	1
Milk chocolate candy, plain	1 oz	145	16	2
Gelatin dessert, prepared	½ cup	70	17	2
Popsicle	1	70	18	0
Pudding, chocolate, instant, from mix	½ cup	155	27	4
Pudding, tapioca, from mix	½ cup	145	25	4
Pudding, vanilla, cooked, from mix	½ cup	145	25	4
Honey	1 tbsp	65	17	0
Jams and preserves	1 tbsp	55	14	0
Sugar, white, granulated	1 tbsp	45	12	0
	1 pkt	25	6	0
Syrup, chocolate flavored, thin	2 tbsp	85	22	1
Table syrup (corn and maple)	2 tbsp	122	32	0

Vegetables

Name	Amount	Calories	Carbohydrate	Protein
Alfalfa seeds, sprouted, raw	1 cup	10	1	1

Name	Amount	Calories	Carbohydrate	Protein
Artichokes, globe, cooked, drained	1	55	12	3
Asparagus, cooked from raw, drained, cut	1 cup	45	8	5
Bean sprouts, mung, cooked, drained	1 cup	25	5	3
Beets, cooked, drained, diced	1 cup	55	11	2
Beet greens, cooked, drained	1 cup	40	8	4
Black-eyed peas, immature, raw, cooked	1 cup	180	30	13
Broccoli, raw	1 spear	40	8	4
Broccoli, cooked from raw, drained	1 spear	50	10	5
	1 cup	45	9	5
Brussels sprouts, cooked from raw, cooked	1 cup	60	13	4
Cabbage, common, cooked, drained	1 cup	30	7	1
Cabbage, common, raw	1 cup	15	4	1
Carrots, cooked from raw	1 cup	70	16	2
Carrots, raw, grated	1 cup	45	11	1
Carrots, raw, whole	1	30	7	1
Cauliflower, raw	1 cup	25	5	2
Cauliflower, cooked from raw	1 cup	30	6	2
Celery, pascal type, raw, stalk	1	5	1	0
Collards, cooked from frozen	1 cup	60	12	5
Collards, cooked from raw	1 cup	25	5	2
Corn, canned, whole kernels, white, no salt	1 cup	165	41	5
Corn, cooked from raw, yellow	1 ear	85	19	3

Name	Amount	Calories	Carbohydrate	Protein
Cucumber with peel	6 slices	5	1	0
Eggplant, cooked, steamed	1 cup	25	6	1
Endive, curly, raw	1 cup	10	2	1
Kale, cooked from raw	1 cup	40	7	2
Kohlrabi, cooked, drained	1 cup	50	11	3
Lettuce, butterhead, raw, head	1	20	4	2
Lettuce, crisp head, raw, pieces	1 cup	5	1	1
Lettuce, loose leaf	1 cup	10	2	1
Mushrooms, cooked, drained	1 cup	40	8	3
Mushrooms, raw	1 cup	20	3	1
Okra pods, cooked	8	25	6	2
Onions, raw, chopped	1 cup	55	12	2
Onions, raw, cooked, drained	1 cup	60	13	2
Onions, raw, sliced	1 cup	40	8	1
Onions, spring, raw	6	10	2	1
Parsnips, cooked, drained	1 cup	125	30	2
Peas, edible pod, cooked, drained	1 cup	65	11	5
Peas, green, frozen cooked, drained	1 cup	125	23	8
Peppers, sweet, red or green, raw	1	20	4	1
Potatoes, baked, flesh only	1	145	34	3
Potatoes, baked with skin	1	220	51	5
Potatoes, French fried, frozen, fried	10	160	20	2
Potatoes, French fried, frozen, oven baked	10	110	17	2
Potatoes, mashed, from dehydrated	1 cup	235	32	4
Pumpkin, cooked from raw	1 cup	50	12	2
Radishes, raw	4	5	1	0
Sauerkraut, canned	1 cup	45	10	2

Name	Amount	Calories	Carbohydrate	Protein
Seaweed, kelp, raw	1 oz	10	3	0
Snap beans, raw, cooked, drained, green	1 cup	45	10	2
Spinach, cooked from raw, drained	1 cup	40	7	5
Spinach, raw	1 cup	10	2	2
Squash, summer, cooked, drained	1 cup	35	8	2
Squash, winter, baked	1 cup	80	18	2
Sweet potatoes, baked, peeled	1	115	28	2
Sweet potatoes, boiled, without peel	1	160	37	2
Tomato juice, canned, without salt	1 cup	40	10	2
Tomato paste, canned, without salt	1 cup	220	49	10
Tomato puree, canned, without salt	1 cup	105	25	4
Tomato sauce, canned, with salt	1 cup	75	18	3
Tomatoes, canned, S&L, with salt	1 cup	50	10	2
Tomatoes, raw	1	25	5	1
Turnips, cooked, diced	1 cup	30	8	1
Turnip greens, cooked from raw	1 cup	30	6	2
Vegetables, mixed, cooked from frozen	1 cup	105	24	5
Water chestnuts, canned	1 cup	70	17	1

Miscellaneous Items

Baking Products, Spices, Vinegar

Name	Amount	Calories	Carbohydrate	Protein
Baking powder, low sodium	1 tsp	5	1	0
Catsup	1 tbsp	15	4	0

Name	Amount	Calories	Carbohydrate	Protein
Celery seed	1 tsp	10	1	0
Chili powder	1 tsp	10	1	0
Chocolate, bitter or baking	1 oz	145	8	3
Cinnamon	1 tsp	5	2	0
Coconut, raw, pieces	1	160	7	1
Coconut, raw, shredded	1 cup	285	12	3
Curry powder	1 tsp	5	1	0
Garlic powder	1 tsp	10	2	0
Gelatin, dry	1 pkt	25	0	6
Mustard, prepared, yellow	1 tsp	5	0	0
Olives, canned, green	4 med	15	0	0
Olives, canned, ripe, mission	3 small	15	0	0
Onion powder	1 tsp	5	2	0
Oregano	1 tsp	5	1	0
Paprika	1 tsp	5	1	0
Pepper, black	1 tsp	5	1	0
Pickles, cucumber, dill	1	5	1	0
Salt	1 tsp	0	0	0
Vinegar, cider	1 tbsp	0	1	0
Yeast, brewer's, dry	1 tbsp	25	3	3

USDA Department of Agriculture, Agricultural Research Service, 1998.
USDA Nutrient Database for Standard Reference, Release 12. Nutrient Data
Laboratory Home Page, http://www.nal.usda.gov/fnic/foodcomp

Bibliography

Bess, Patti A. *Vegetarian Barbecue & Other Pleasures of the Harvest*. Los Angeles: Lowell House, 1999.

Borushek, Allan. *The Doctor's Pocket Calorie Fat & Carbohydrate Counter*. California: Family Health Publications, 2001.

Brand-Miller, Jennie, Ph.D., Thomas M. S. Wolever, M.D., Ph.D., Stephen Colagiuri, M.D., and Kaye Foster-Powell, M. Nutr. & Diet. *The Glucose Revolution: The Authoritative Guide to the Glycemic Index*. New York: Marlowe & Company, 1999.

Ezrin, Calvin, M.D., and Robert Kowalski. *The Type 2 Diabetes Diet Book*. Los Angeles: Lowell House, 1995.

Ezrin, Calvin, M.D., and Kristen L. Caron, M.A. *Your Fat Can Make You Thin*. Los Angeles: Lowell House, 2000.

Geil, Patti B., M.S., R.D., F.A.D.A., C.D.E. and Lee Ann Holzmeister, R.D., C.D.E. *101 Nutrition Tips for People with Diabetes*. American Diabetes Association, 1999.

Holt, Susanne, H. A., Janette C. Brand-Miller, and Peter Petocz. "An Insulin Index of Foods: The Insulin Demand Generated by 1000-kj

Portions of Common Foods." *American Journal of Clinical Nutrition* 6b (1997): 1264–76.

Heller, Dr. Richard F., Dr. Rachael F. Heller, and Dr. Frederic J. Vagnini. *The Carbohydrate Addict's Healthy Heart Program.* New York: Random House, 1999.

Loring, Gloria. *The Kids, Food and Diabetes Family Cookbook.* Gloria Loring for the Juvenile Diabetes Foundation International, 1991.

Ludwig, David S., et al. "High Glycemic Index Foods, Overeating, and Obesity." *Pediatrics* 103, no. 3 (March 1999): e26ff.

Netzer, Corinne T. *The Complete Book of Food Counts.* New York: Dell Publishing, 1991.

Raloff, J. "The New GI Tracts." *Science News Online* 157, no. 15 (2000): 236.

Soneral, Lois M. *The Type 2 Diabetes Desserts Cookbook.* Los Angeles: Lowell House, 1999.

Index